T0329003

CYCLOSPORA AND CYCLOSPORIASIS

CYCLOSPORA AND CYCLOSPORIASIS
Epidemiology, Diagnosis, Detection, and Control

Long-Xian Zhang
Henan Province Distinguished Professor, Henan Agricultural University, Zhengzhou, China

Rong-Jun Wang
Professor, Henan Agricultural University, Zhengzhou, China

Guang-Hui Zhao
Professor, New Century Talents of Chinese Ministry of Education, Northwest A&F University, Yangling, China

Jun-Qiang Li
Assistant Professor, Henan Agricultural University, Zhengzhou, China

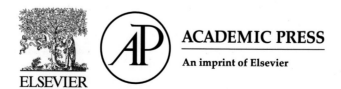

ACADEMIC PRESS
An imprint of Elsevier

ELSEVIER

Academic Press is an imprint of Elsevier
125 London Wall, London EC2Y 5AS, United Kingdom
525 B Street, Suite 1650, San Diego, CA 92101, United States
50 Hampshire Street, 5th Floor, Cambridge, MA 02139, United States
The Boulevard, Langford Lane, Kidlington, Oxford OX5 1GB, United Kingdom

Notices
Knowledge and best practice in this field are constantly changing. As new research and experience
broaden our understanding, changes in research methods, professional practices, or medical
treatment may become necessary.

Practitioners and researchers must always rely on their own experience and knowledge in
evaluating and using any information, methods, compounds, or experiments described herein. In
using such information or methods they should be mindful of their own safety and the safety of
others, including parties for whom they have a professional responsibility.

To the fullest extent of the law, neither the Publisher nor the authors, contributors, or editors,
assume any liability for any injury and/or damage to persons or property as a matter of products
liability, negligence or otherwise, or from any use or operation of any methods, products,
instructions, or ideas contained in the material herein.

Library of Congress Cataloging-in-Publication Data
A catalog record for this book is available from the Library of Congress

British Library Cataloguing-in-Publication Data
A catalogue record for this book is available from the British Library

ISBN: 978-0-12-821616-3

For information on all Academic Press publications
visit our website at https://www.elsevier.com/books-and-journals

Publisher: Andre Gerhard Wolff
Acquisitions Editor: Kattie Washington
Editorial Project Manager: Ruby Smith
Production Project Manager: Maria Bernard
Cover Designer: Christian J. Bilbow

Typeset by SPi Global, India

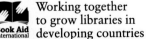

Working together
to grow libraries in
developing countries

www.elsevier.com • www.bookaid.org

Contents

Preface

Globally, there are nearly 1.7 billion reported cases of diarrheal disease every year, and its socioeconomic burden on health services has been estimated at 72.8 million disability-adjusted life years annually. Enteric protozoan parasites are known to be among the major contributors to the diarrheal disease load, and *Cyclospora cayetanensis* (*C. cayetanensis*) is an important global protozoan pathogen in humans, typically causing prolonged diarrhea accompanied by anorexia, malaise, nausea, and cramping, among other symptoms. Notably, several large outbreaks of cyclosporiasis have been documented in developed countries, and *C. cayetanensis* infections are also most commonly reported in developing countries or in endemic areas. Human *C. cayetanensis* infection has been reported in over 56 countries worldwide, and 13 of these have recorded cyclosporiasis outbreaks, resulting in significant economic losses and public health concerning. Although treatment with trimethoprim-sulfamethoxazole (TMP-SMX) has proven effective for cyclosporiasis, other antiparasitic agents should be considered for patients having sulfur drug intolerance or resistance. Furthermore, no vaccine candidates are available for cyclosporiasis.

Fortunately, great progresses were achieved in last decades in epidemiology, diagnosis, detection, and control of *C. cayetanensis* infection and cyclosporiasis. Although exact transmission routs of *Cyclospora* are still not clear, contaminated water and various types of fresh food or produce have been reported responsible for most large outbreaks. Protocols for diagnosis as early as possible to identify *Cyclospora* infection in human populations and to trace the source of transmission would be the best approach for the control of cyclosporiasis. The whole genome of *C. cayetanensis* had been sequenced, and there have been recent improvements in detection methods and therapeutic interventions for cyclosporiasis. More than 1000 papers have been published about *Cyclospora*. Numerous studies of *Cyclospora* infection among travelers, patients with immune deficiency, diarrheal or asymptomatic patients, and endemic area residents have been conducted and reported. There are few books on the biological characteristics, clinical features, epidemiology, detection methods, and treatment of *C. cayetanensis* to assess some risk factors for human infection with this foodborne pathogen. However, in most of these published books, the *Cyclospora* spp. and *Cyclospora cayetanensis* are embodied only as one of the chapters.

For this, this book presents the detail known information about the *Cyclospora* spp. and *Cyclospora cayetanensis*.

We hope that the book would provide support for scholars in microbiology, parasitology, and epidemiology to understand the *Cyclospora* and cyclosporiasis, for clinicians to rapidly diagnose and treat the infection of cyclosporosis, for the importers/exporters and customs officers for dealing with regulation of transporting fresh products, and for the public health and food safety officials to assess the hazard of *C. cayetanensis* trans-regional transmissions.

Acknowledgments

This study was financially supported, in part, by the Zhongyuan One Thousand Talents Program of China (19CZ0122), National Major Scientific and Technological Special Projects of China (2012ZX10004220-011), National Major Scientific and Technological Special Project of China (2008ZX10004-011), and Major Public Welfare Scientific Research Projects in Henan Province, China (81100912300).

We are thankful to the research platform of National Joint International Research Center for Animal Immunology (Zhengzhou, China) and International Joint Research Laboratory for Zoonotic Diseases of Henan, China (Zhengzhou, China).

We are grateful to Prof. Lihua Xiao (South China Agricultural University), Prof. Ronald Fayer (United States Department of Agriculture), Prof. Guan Zhu (Texas A&M University), and Prof. Haining Shi (Harvard University) for their critical review on scientific research ideas and technical data. We also extend our thanks to all the scholars who have communicated and discussed with us under this topic.

CHAPTER 1

Taxonomy and biology

Contents

1.1 Introduction

The species of the genus *Cyclospora*, *Cyclospora glomericola*, was first described in the millipede Glomeris (Diplopoda) by Aimé Schneider in 1881 (Ortega and Sanchez, 2010). The human cyclosporosis pathogenic organism was first described in three patients in Papua New Guinea (Ashford et al., 1979), and named as *Cyclospora cayetanensis* by Ortega et al. in 1994 (Ortega and Sanchez, 2010). As of today, 22 named *Cyclospora* species have been identified in the humans and various animals, including vipers, moles, myriapodes, rodents, and monkeys (McAllister et al., 2018; Li et al., 2020). Besides, some *Cyclospora*-like organisms, none of which got valid species name, have also been described in dogs, cattle, chickens, rats/house mice, birds, monkeys, shellfish, etc., and even in environmental samples (Li et al., 2020).

Microscopically, *Cyclospora* oocysts are usually visible with modified Ziehl-Neelsen acid-fast staining (Clarke and McIntyre, 1996; Zhou et al., 2011). Furthermore, the oocyst wall autofluorescences under fluorescence microscopy, which is an important characteristic of *Cyclospora* parasite (Zhou et al., 2011). The oocysts of *Cyclospora* morphologically slightly differ by species under microscope and are mostly spheroidal, subspheroidal, ovoid, or ellipsoidal in forms. When sporulated, each oocyst has two ovoid sporocysts that in turn contain two sporozoites each (Ortega and Sanchez, 2010).

Taxonomically, *Cyclospora* belongs to the Apicomplexa subphylum, Coccidiasina subclass, Eimeriidae family, and *Cyclospora* genus (Ortega and Sanchez, 2010). Phylogenetic analysis had revealed that human–associated *Cyclospora* is closely related to members of the genus *Eimeria* (Relman et al., 1996; Liu et al., 2016). The life cycle-related infection of *Cyclospora* is similar to that of the most of the other Apicomplexan intestinal parasite that mainly occurs via the fecal-oral transmission route (Almeria et al., 2019). The presence of asexual and sexual stages in the same host suggests that the life cycle of the microorganism can be completed within one host (Ortega et al., 1997).

1.2 History of discovery and research

1.2.1 *Cyclospora* detected in animals

The species of the genus *Cyclospora*, *C. glomericola*, was described in the millipede Glomeris (Diplopoda) by Aimé Schneider in 1881 and, to date, appears to be the only species encountered in an invertebrate host (Lainson, 2005).

In 1870, Eimer noted the presence of a parasite with Cyclosporan morphology in the intestine of the mole Talpa europaea, but did not propose any name for the parasite. In 1902, Schaudinn named the parasite *Cyclospora caryolytica* and gave a full description of its life cycle. Tanabe (1938) later described the development of what he considered to be the same species in another mole referred to as *Mogera wogura coreana* from Japan (Lainson, 2005).

There followed a succession of descriptions of other *Cyclospora* species in reptiles, snakes, and monkeys, most with intracytoplasmic development in epithelial cells of the intestine (Table 1.1). However, Pellérdy and Tanyi (1968) described the oocysts of a second species in the European mole and named it *Cyclospora talpae*. They observed the parasitic microgamonts and macrogamonts in the liver, and, in 1990, Mohamed and Molyneux showed that these sexual stages developed within the nucleus of the bile-duct epithelial cells. Duszynski and Wattam (1988) redescribed the oocysts of *C. talpae* in European mole (*T. europaea*) from England and, in addition, noted that some oocysts were present which differed from those of *C. talpae* in minor details (principally in size). Whether or not they belonged to another species of *Cyclospora* has not been decided yet. Ford and Duszynski (1988) turned their attention to fecal samples from other members of the Insectivora and encountered three further species of *Cyclospora*. *Cyclospora megacephali* was described in the "eastern mole" *Scalopus aquaticus*, and both *Cyclospora ashtabulensis* and *Cyclospora parascalopi* in the "hairy-tailed mole" *Parascalops breweri*. The site of development in these animals was not ascertained. Ford et al. (1990) gave the name *Cyclospora angimurinensis* to oocysts they found in the feces of the heteromyid rodent *Chaetodipus hispidus* from the United States and Northern Mexico. Once again, the site of endogenous development was not determined (Lainson, 2005).

Four *Cyclospora* species have been described in nonhuman primates: *Cyclospora cercopitheci* in vervet monkeys (*Cercopithecus aethiops*), *Cyclospora colobi* in colobus monkeys (*Colobus guereza*), and *Cyclospora papionis* in olive baboons (*Papio anubis*) in 1999 (Eberhard et al., 1999); and *Cyclospora macacae* in rhesus monkeys (*Macaca mulatta*) in 2015 (Li et al., 2015). In 2018, two more species namely *Cyclospora duszynskii* and *Cyclospora yatesi* have been characterized in moles (*S. aquaticus*) (McAllister et al., 2018). Thus, 22 valid *Cyclospora* species have been described in humans and various animals till to date.

Table 1.1 The type host, oocyst morphology, and endogenous stages of reported *Cyclospora* spp.

Species names	Named by, Year	Type host (scientific name)	Oocyst morphology	Oocyst size (μm)	Shape index (L:W)	Endogenous stages
C. glomericola	Schneider, 1881	Glomeris sp.	–	25.0–36.0×9.0–10.0	–	Not described, oocysts in lumen of gut
C. caryolytica	Schaudinn, 1902	Mogera wogura	–	18.0×12.5	–	Intranuclear in epithelial cells of small and large intestine
C. viperae	Phisalix, 1923	Vipera aspis	–	16.8×10.5	–	Intranuclear in epithelial cells of small and large intestine
C. babaulti	Phisalix, 1924	Vipera berus	–	17.0×10.0	–	Intranuclear in epithelial cells of small and large intestine
C. scinci	Phisalix, 1924	Scincus officinalis	–	10.0×7.0	–	Intranuclear in epithelial cells of small and large intestine
C. tropidonoti	Phisalix, 1924	Natrix stolata Lacepede	–	17.0×10.0	–	Intranuclear in epithelial cells of small and large intestine
C. zamenis	Phisalix, 1924	Coluber viridiflatus Lacepede	–	17.0×10.0	–	Intranuclear in epithelial cells of small and large intestine
C. niniae	Lainson, 1965	Ninia sebae	–	14.6×13.3	–	Intranuclear in epithelial cells of small and large intestine

Species	Reference	Host	Oocyst shape	Oocyst size	Shape index	Endogenous development site
C. talpae	Pellérdy and Tanyi, 1968	*Talpa europaea*	Ellipsoidal	12.0–19.0×6.0–13.0 (mean 14.3×9.6)	1.2–1.9 (mean 1.5)	Intranuclear in epithelial cells of bile ducts and capillary sinusoids of the liver
Cyclospora sp.	Duszynski and Wattam, 1988	*Hemidactylus frenatus*	Subspheroidal to ellipsoidal	10.0–14.0×6.0–12.0 (mean 12.7×8.9)	1.2–1.9 (mean 1.4)	Not ascertained
C. megacephali	Ford and Duszynski, 1988	*Scalopus aquaticus*	Subspheroidal	14.0–21.0×12.0–18.0 (mean 18.5×15.7)	1.1–1.4 (mean 1.2)	Not ascertained
C. ashtabulensis	Ford and Duszynski, 1989	*Parascalops breweri*	Subspheroidal to ellipsoidal	14.0–23.0×11.0–19.0 (mean 18.0×14.3)	1.1–1.7 (mean 1.3)	Not ascertained
C. parascalopi	Ford and Duszynski, 1989	*Parascalops breweri*	Ellipsoidal	13.0–20.0×11.0–20.0 (16.5×13.6 μm)	1.0–1.5 (mean 1.2)	Not ascertained
C. angimurinensis	Ford et al., 1990	*Chaetodipus hispidus*	Subspheroidal	19.0–24.0×16.0–22.0 (mean 21.9×19.3)	1.1–1.3 (mean 1.1)	Not ascertained
C. cayetanensis	Ortega et al., 1994	*Homo sapiens*	Spheroidal	7.7–9.9 (mean 8.6)	1.0–1.1	Intracytoplasmic in epithelial cells of the intestine
C. cercopitheci	Eberhard et al., 1999	*Cercopithecus aethiops*	Spherical	8.0–10.0 (mean 9.2)	1.0–1.1	Not ascertained

Continued

Table 1.1 The type host, oocyst morphology, and endogenous stages of reported Cyclospora spp.—cont'd

Species names	Named by, Year	Type host (scientific name)	Oocyst morphology	Oocyst size (μm)	Shape index (L:W)	Endogenous stages
C. colobi	Eberhard et al., 1999	Colobus guereza	Spherical	8.0–9.0 μm (mean 8.3 μm)	1.0–1.1	Not ascertained
C. papionis	Eberhard et al., 1999	Papio anubis	Spherical	8–10 (mean 8.8)	1.0–1.1	Not ascertained
C. schneider	Lainson, 2005	Anilius scytale scytale	Ovoid to subspherical	15.1–25.7×13.8–20.1 (mean 19.8×16.6)	1–1.3 (mean 1.2)	Intracytoplasmic in epithelial cells of the intestine
C. macacae	Li et al., 2015	Macaca mulatta	Spherical	8.49±0.55×8.49±0.49	1.02	Not ascertained
C. duszynskii	McAllister et al., 2018	Scalopus aquaticus	Subspheroidal	10.0–12.0×9.0–11.0 (mean 11.4×10.0)	1.0–1.2 (mean 1.1)	Unknown; oocysts recovered from feces
C. yatesi	McAllister et al., 2018	Scalopus aquaticus	Subspheroidal to ovoidal	12.0–18.0×10.0–17.0 (mean 17.0×15.2)	1.0–1.2 (mean 1.1)	Unknown; oocysts recovered from feces

1.2.2 *Cyclospora* detected in humans

In 1979, Ashford published first report recording the presence of what were most probably oocysts of *Cyclospora* in the feces of three patients in Papua New Guinea, two of whom were suffering from diarrhea (Ashford, 1979). The oocysts contained two sporocysts, but Ashford was unable to identify the parasite to generic level due to difficulties in determining the number of sporozoites in the sporocysts. This important finding, strangely overlooked in much of the literature, was followed by a series of publications on similar findings in patients, most of whom were suffering from acute "traveler's diarrhea" acquired in areas with poor standards of hygiene or in immunocompromised (AIDS) patients (Lainson, 2005). Long et al. (1991) proposed the term "cyanobacterium-like bodies" (CLB) for the cysts because of a superficial ultrastructural resemblance to unicellular members of the blue-green algae. Bendall et al. indicated the coccidial nature of the cyanobacterium-like bodies, illustrated by photomicrographs of the sporulated oocysts containing two sporocysts. The name *C. cayetanensis* was later proposed by these authors in an abstract of this presentation, although Ashford et al. (1993) questioned the validity of the name in view of what they considered to be an inadequate written description of the parasite and the absence of illustrations (Ortega and Sanchez, 2010). Subsequently, Ortega et al. (1994) described the light and electron microscopic morphology of the oocysts in detail and the specific name *C. cayetanensis* now remains in firm usage (Lainson, 2005).

There were some scattered reports before 1990s that claimed the presence of *Cyclospora* oocysts in the feces of patients, such as patients from Haiti and Peru during 1983–85, American travelers returning from Haiti and Mexico in 1986, British travelers who became ill in Nepal in 1989, and travelers and foreign residents in Nepal in 1993 (Herwaldt, 2000); the identity of the organisms was uncertain at that time, and most probably were *Cyclospora* oocysts. *C. cayetanensis* has received greater attention since the first outbreak of diarrheal illness associated with *Cyclospora* in the United States in 1990 (Huang et al., 1995). In 1996, more than 1400 cases of cyclosporiasis have been reported in the United States and Canada (Herwaldt and Ackers, 1997). Since then, very large studies of *Cyclospora* infection among travelers, patients with immune deficiency, diarrheal patients, and asymptomatic individuals have been conducted and reported, as have studies addressing detection methods and treatment measures for *Cyclospora*. The most recent large outbreaks were documented in 2013 and 2018 concerning

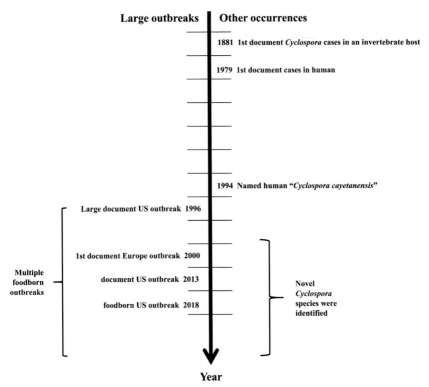

Fig. 1.1 A time line of the increasing activity and expanding knowledge about the *Cyclospora* organism (*C. cayetanensis*). *(Adapted from Herwaldt, B.L., 2000. Cyclospora cayetanensis: a review, focusing on the outbreaks of cyclosporiasis in the 1990s. Clin. Infect. Dis. 31, 1040–1057.)*

multistate foodborne cyclosporiasis outbreaks in the United States (Abanyie et al., 2015; Casillas et al., 2018). A time line of the increasing activity and expanding knowledge about the *Cyclospora* organism (*C. cayetanensis*) are shown in Fig. 1.1.

1.3 Morphology

Cyclospora species are found in reptiles and mammals, and the morphology of the parasitic oocysts differs by species under light microscopy (Table 1.1). However, they mostly have a spheroidal, subspheroidal, ovoid, or ellipsoidal form. When sporulated, each oocyst has two ovoid sporocysts that in turn contain two sporozoites each (Ortega and Sanchez, 2010).

By light microscopy, it is clearly difficult to determine the number of sporozoites in a sporocyst of an oocyst as small as that of *C. cayetanensis*

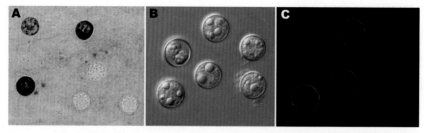

Fig. 1.2 Morphology of *C. cayetanensis* oocysts under microscopy. Oocysts in stool smears stained with modified acid-fast stain under light microscopy; two oocysts are stained with different intensities (A); under differential interference contrast microscopy of wet mounts, a partially sporulated oocyst can be seen (B); epifluorescence microscopy with a 330–380-nm UV excitation filter (C). *(Reference to Zhou, Y., Lv, B., Wang, Q., Wang, R., Jian, F., Zhang, L., Ning, C., Fu, K., Wang, Y., Qi, M., Yao, H., Zhao, J., Zhang, X., Sun, Y., Shi, K., Arrowood, M.J., Xiao, L., 2011. Prevalence and molecular characterization of Cyclospora cayetanensis, Henan, China. Emerg. Infect. Dis. 17, 1887–1890.)*

(diameter 8.6 μm), and other *Cyclospora* species of similar size may well have been erroneously assigned to the genus *Isospora* or *Sarcocystis*. However, due to the much larger size of the oocysts of both *Cyclospora niniae* and *Cyclospora schneideri* (14.6×13.3 and 19.8×16.6, respectively), it has not been difficult to determine the dizoic nature of their sporocysts, particularly when they are seen in an end-on position.

   C. cayetanensis oocysts under light microscopy have a spheroid shape, 8–10 μm in diameter, with indistinguishable protoplasm. When sporulated, each oocyst has two ovoid sporocysts that in turn contain two sporozoites each (Fig. 1.2). *C. cayetanensis* oocysts are stained differently with modified Ziehl–Neelsen acid-fast stain: some stained dark red with a mottled appearance, some stained pink, while others not stained at all and appear as nonrefractile glassy spheres against the blue-green background (Clarke and McIntyre, 1996; Zhou et al., 2011). Autofluorescence renders *C. cayetanensis* oocysts easily visible in clinical samples under epifluorescence microscopy, with blue fluorescence under an ultraviolet filter of 330–380 nm, and green fluorescence under an ultraviolet filter of 450–490 nm (Zhou et al., 2011).

1.4 Taxonomy

Cyclospora is closely related to members of the *Eimeria* genus (Relman et al., 1996; Liu et al., 2016), and *Cyclospora* genus belongs to the Apicomplexa subphylum, Coccidiasina subclass, Eimeriidae family, and *Cyclospora* genus (Ortega and Sanchez, 2010). As of today, 22 valid species of *Cyclospora* have been described in snakes, moles, myriapodes, rodents, monkeys, and humans (Lainson, 2005; Li et al., 2015; McAllister et al., 2018).

1.4.1 *Cyclospora glomericola* (Schneider, 1881; Lainson, 2005)

Description: Oocysts of 25.0–36.0×9.0–10.0 µm in size.

Type host: *Glomeris* sp.

Site of infection/endogenous stages: Not described, oocysts in lumen of gut.

Named by: Schneider in 1881.

Remarks: *C. glomericola* was first described in the millipede *Glomeris* (Diplopoda) by Aimé Schneider in 1881 and, to date, appears to be the only species encountered in an invertebrate host.

1.4.2 *Cyclospora caryolytica* (Schaudinn, 1902; Tanabe, 1938)

Description: Oocysts of 18.0×12.5 µm in size.

Type host: *T. europaea, Mogera wogura coreana* (Insectivora: Talpidae).

Type locality: Japan.

Site of infection/endogenous stages: Intranuclear in epithelial cells of small and large intestines. Asexual and sexual stages of *C. caryolytica* both in the small and in the large intestine of the mole, where they develop within the nucleus of the epithelial cells.

Named by: Schaudinn in 1902.

Remarks: Previously, Eimer (1870) had noted the presence of a parasite with cyclosporan morphology in the intestine of the mole *T. europaea*, but gave it no name, and it remained for Schaudinn (1902) to give a full description of the life cycle of this parasite, which he named *C. caryolytica*. Tanabe (1938) later described the development of what he considered to be the same species in another mole referred to as *M. wogura coreana* from Japan.

1.4.3 *Cyclospora viperae* (Phisalix, 1923; Lainson, 2005)

Description: Oocysts of 16.8×10.5 µm in size.

Type host: *Vipera aspis* (Reptilia: Ophidia).

Other natural hosts: *Coluber scalaris, Coronella austriaca, Natrix viperinus.*

Site of infection/endogenous stages: Intracytoplasmic in epithelial cells of the intestine.

Named by: Phisalix in 1923.

Remarks: Phisalix made a number of revisions to her measurements of the oocysts of *C. viperae*, but on the basis of her final measurements of 16.8 × 10.5 μm, they are considered substantially smaller than those of *C. schneideri*, as are those of *Cyclospora babaulti*, *Cyclospora tropidonoti*, and *Cyclospora zamenis* (17.0 × 10.0 μm). Without cross-infection experiments, the host specificity of ophidian *Cyclospora* species remains uncertain, but the wide zoological difference and wide geographical separation of the European colubrids and vipers makes it most unlikely that *C. schneideri* is conspecific with any one of the species described by Phisalix. Based on the similarity of the oocysts of the four species of *Cyclospora* named by Phisalix (Lainson, 1965), it is commented and suggested that **C. babaulti, C. tropidonoti,** and *C. zamenis* might be synonyms of **C. viperae**. Duszynski et al. (1999) partly agreed with this suggestion and listed **C. babaulti** as a synonym of **C. viperae** and **C. tropidonoti** as a synonym of **C. zamenis**.

1.4.4 *Cyclospora scinci* (Phisalix, 1924; Lainson, 2005)

Description: Oocysts of 10.0 × 7.0 μm in size.
    Type host: *Scincus officinalis* (Reptilia, Squamata, Scincidae).
    Site of infection/endogenous stages: Intracytoplasmic in epithelial cells of the intestine.
    Named by: Phisalix in 1924.

1.4.5 *Cyclospora zamenis* (Phisalix, 1924; Lainson, 2005)

Description: Oocysts of 17.0 × 10.0 μm in size.
    Type host: *Coluber viridiflavus viridiflavus* (Reptilia: Ophidia).
    Site of infection/endogenous stages: Intracytoplasmic in epithelial cells of intestine.
    Named by: Phisalix in 1924.

1.4.6 *Cyclospora tropidonoti* (Phisalix, 1924; Lainson, 2005)

Description: Oocysts of 17.0 × 10.0 μm in size.
    Type host: *Natrix natrix*, *Natrix stolata* (Reptilia: Ophidia).
    Site of infection/endogenous stages: Intracytoplasmic in epithelial cells of the intestine.
    Named by: Phisalix in 1924.

1.4.7 *Cyclospora babaulti* (Phisalix, 1924; Lainson, 2005)

Description: Oocysts of 17.0 × 10.0 μm in size.
    Type host: *Vipera berus* (Reptilia: Ophidia).

Site of infection/endogenous stages: Intracytoplasmic in epithelial cells of the intestine.

Named by: Phisalix in 1924.

1.4.8 *Cyclospora niniae* (Lainson, 1965)

Description: Oocysts of 14.6×13.3 μm in size, contain a conspicuous polar body, fragile oocyst wall, a number of sporocysts, and possess a modest Stieda body.

Type host: *Ninia sebae sebae* (Reptilia: Ophidia).

Site of infection/endogenous stages: Intracytoplasmic in epithelial cells of intestine.

Named by: Lainson in 1965.

1.4.9 *Cyclospora ashtabulensis* (Ford and Duszynski, 1989)

Description: Oocyst subspheroidal to ellipsoidal with thick wall (> 1.0) composed of two layers: outer layer rough and inner layer smooth. Polar body, oocyst residuum, and micropyle absent. Sporulated oocysts (n = 23) 14.0–23.0×11.0–19.0 μm (mean 18.0×14.3 μm) with L:W ratio 1.1–1.7 (mean 1.3); sporocysts (n = 23) ovoid, 8.0–14.0×5.0–9.0 (mean 11.6×7.2 μm) with L:W ratio 1.2–2.0 (mean 1.6); membranous material between sporocysts appears to hold them together; Stieda body present as crescent-shaped cap covering rounded end of sporocyst, but sub- and para-Stieda bodies absent; sporocyst residuum of several large globules that may obscure sporozoites or present as a compact mass.

Type host: *Parascalop breweri* (Bachman, 1842).

Type locality: Ashtabula County, Ohio.

Prevalence: Found in 7 of the 16 (44%) fecal samples of *P. breweri*, all of them from Ashtabula County, Ohio.

Site of infection: Unknown, oocysts collected from feces.

Material deposited: Phototypes of oocysts in the USNM Parasite Collection No. 80590. Host skin, skull, skeleton, chromosomes, tissue culture cells, and blood in the Museum of Southwestern Biology, Division of Mammalogy, NK 3121 (male), K. McBee #120, June 29, 1980, MSB #43419.

Etymology: The species name is derived from the name of the county where the host was collected.

Remarks: Oocysts of this species resemble those of *C. megacephali* (Ford and Duszynski, 1988) described from the eastern mole, *S. aquaticus* (Linnaeus, 1758), because both have an unusual crescent-like Stieda body

(Ford and Duszynski, 1988). It differs from *C. megacephali* by having oocysts that lack polar bodies, have rough outer walls (vs smooth), and are slightly small (18.0×14.0 vs 19.0×16.0 μm). The sporocysts of *C. ashtabulensis* are less elongate (12.0×7.0 μm) than those of *C. megacephali* (15.0×7.0 μm) and thus have a smaller shape index (1.6 vs 2.1); they also do not have a pointed end opposite Stieda body.

1.4.10 *Cyclospora talpae* (Duszynski and Wattam, 1988)

Description: Oocyst ellipsoidal with thin wall composed of two layers: outer layer smooth, ~⅓ of total wall thickness; micropyle, oocyst residuum, and polar body absent; sporulated oocysts (*n*=71) 12.0–19.0×6.0–13.0 μm (mean 14.3×9.6 μm); L:W ratio 1.2–1.9 (mean 1.5); sporocysts ovoidal, pointed at one end, 6.0–13.0×4.0–8.0 μm (mean 9.4×5.7 μm); L:W ratio 1.3–2.1 (mean 1.7); Stieda and substieda bodies present, about equal in width, but para-Stieda body absent; sporocyst residuum of many large, spherical globules.

Type locality: England (Avon, Norfolk, Surrey).

Prevalence: Found in 21 of the 33 (63.6%) fecal samples of *T. europaea* from which sporulated oocysts were recovered.

Site of infection. Unknown. Oocysts recovered from feces.

Named by: Duszynski and Wattam in 1988.

Remarks: The oocysts described by Duszynski and Wattam differed in several respects from those described by Pellérdy and Tanyi from *T. europaea* from Hungary: (1) the sporulated oocysts were generally ellipsoidal and were not "asymmetrical bodies, tapering toward both ends" and (2) the sporocysts had a substieda body about the same width as the Stieda body, but this structure was seen only when carefully viewed with Nomarski Interference Contrast (NIC) microscopy, which Pellérdy and Tanyi did not use. The photomicrograph published by Pellérdy and Tanyi, however, showed an oocyst that indicated the same species described differently by the two groups of researchers. The attempts by Duszynski and Wattam to induce sporozoites to excyst in order to count sporozoites per sporocyst were unsuccessful. However, the observations and photomicrographs suggested the presence of only two sporozoites per sporocyst.

1.4.11 *Cyclospora* sp. (Duszynski and Wattam, 1988)

Description: Oocyst subspherical to ellipsoidal with thin wall (≤1.0) composed of two layers: outer layer smooth, ~ ⅓ of total thickness; micropyle, oocyst residuum, and polar body absent; sporulated oocysts (*n*=50)

10.0–14.0×6.0–12.0 μm (mean 12.7×8.9 μm); L:W ratio 1.2–1.9 (mean 1.4); sporocysts ovoidal, distinctly pointed at one end, 6–10×4–6 μm (mean 8.6×5.3 μm); L:W ratio 1.3–2.0 (mean 1.6); Stieda and substieda bodies present, about equal in width, but para-Stieda body absent; sporocyst residuum of 2–6 large, spheroidal globules.

Type locality: England (Avon, Norfolk, Surrey).

Prevalence: Found in 21 of the 33 (63.6%) fecal samples of *T. europaea* from which sporulated oocysts were recovered.

Site of infection: Unknown. Oocysts recovered from feces.

Named by: Duszynski and Wattam in 1988.

Remarks: Oocysts of this form most closely resemble those which were identified as *C. talpae*, but differ by having generally smaller oocysts; and a Stieda body that seems more pointed than blunt; and fewer globules that make up the sporocyst residuum. Although both oocyst ($P \leq .01$) and sporocyst ($P \leq .05$) length and width measurements differ significantly between the two forms and there is a shape difference between their Stieda bodies, these factors may be part of the normal variation in the oocysts of this coccidium. Until other evidence is available either to combine these forms or name this one as new, it is preferred to bring this information to the attention of other workers in the field. Attempts to induce sporozoites to excyst from this form were also unsuccessful. Duszynski and Wattam (1988) redescribed the oocysts of *C. talpae* in *T. europaea* from England and, in addition, noted that some oocysts were present which differed from those of *C. talpae* in minor details (principally in size). Whether or not they belonged to another species of *Cyclospora* has not been decided yet.

1.4.12 *Cyclospora megacephali* (Ford and Duszynski, 1988)

Description: Oocyst subspheroidal with thin wall (~1.0) composed of two layers of equal thickness: outer layer smooth; micropyle and oocyst residuum absent; polar body of 3–5 small granules or one larger globule, but usually obscured by sporocysts; sporulated oocysts ($n = 34$) 14.0–21.0×12.0–18.0 μm (mean 18.5×15.7 μm) with L:W ratio 1.1–1.4 (mean 1.2); sporocysts ($n = 34$), 11.0–17.0×6.0–9.0 μm (mean 15.0×7.2 μm) with L:W ratio 1.7–2.4 (mean 2.1); Stieda body present as large cap, covering rounded end of sporocyst; end of sporocyst opposite Stieda body slightly pointed; sub- and para-Stieda bodies absent; sporocyst residuum a compact mass of large clumped globules; sporozoites with 1–2 refractile bodies usually visible.

Type host: *S. aquaticus* (Linnaeus, 1758), Museum of South- western Biology, Division of Mammalogy, NK 2034 (female), J. A. Cook #239, May 19, 1980, MSB #42353.

Type locality: Motley Co., TX.

Prevalence: Found in 4 of the 13 (31%) fecal samples of *S. aquaticus*.

Site of infection: Unknown, oocysts recovered from feces.

Etymology: The species name is derived from *mega* and *cephali* to emphasize the large size of the Stieda body on the sporocysts.

Named by: Ford and Duszynski in 1988.

Remarks: Oocysts of *C. megacephali*, because of the unique shape of its sporocysts with their large, cap-like Stieda bodies, do not resemble any previous cyclosporans. Oocysts were 709–2032 days old when measured.

1.4.13 *Cyclospora parascalopi* (Ford and Duszynski, 1989)

Description: Oocyst generally subspheroidal with thick wall (> 1.0) composed of two layers: outer layer striated, slightly sculptured; inner layer smooth. Oocyst residuum, micropyle, and polar body absent. Sporulated oocysts ($n=62$) 13.0–20.0×11.0–20.0 μm (mean 16.5×13.6 μm) with L:W ratio 1.0–1.5 (mean 1.2); sporocysts (n = 62) ovoid, 8.0–14.0×5.0–8.0 μm (mean 11.1×6.9 μm) with L:W ratio 1.2–2.0 (mean 1.6); prominent, thick Stieda body present, but sub- and para-Stieda bodies absent; sporocyst residuum a single large sphere.

Type host: *P. breweri* (Bachman, 1842).

Type locality: Ashtabula County, Ohio.

Prevalence: Found in 8 of the 16 (50%) fecal samples of *P. breweri*, including 2 of 9 (22%) from Franklin County, Massachusetts, and 6 of 7 (86%) from Ashtabula County, Ohio.

Site of infection: Unknown, oocysts collected from feces.

Material deposited: Phototypes of oocysts in the USNM Parasite Collection No. 80591. Host skin, skull, skeleton, chromosomes, and tissue (heart, kidney, liver) in the Museum of Southwestern Biology, Division of Mammalogy, NK 3109 (female), R. M. Sullivan #509, June 28, 1980, MSB #43418.

Etymology: The species name is derived from the generic name of the host.

Remarks: Oocysts of this species do not resemble those from any species previously described from insectivores, although they are similar in size to those of *C. megacephali* from *S. aquaticus* (Ford and Duszynski, 1988) and to those of *C. ashtabulensis*.

1.4.14 *Cyclospora angimurinensis* (Ford, 1990)

Description: Oocyst subspheroidal with thin wall composed of two layers of equal thickness: outer layer smooth; micropyle absent; oocyst residuum as 3–4 clumped globes of different sizes; 1 polar body present; sporulated oocysts ($n=52$), 19.0–24.0×16.0–22.0 μm (mean 21.9×19.3 μm) with L:W ratio 1.1–1.3 (mean 1.1); sporocysts ($n=51$) lemon-shaped, 9.0–15.0×8.0–11.0 μm (mean 11.9×9.5 μm) with L:W ratio 1.1–1.5 (mean 1.25); Stieda body present, but sub- and para-Stieda bodies are absent; sporocyst residuum of small granules, either compact or dispersed; sporozoites with large posterior refractile body.

Type host: *Chaetodipus hispidus hispidus* (Baird, 1858), hispid pocket mouse.

Type locality: USA., Texas, Somervell County, 0.4 km NNE Nemo off county road 407.

Prevalence: Found in 1 of the 20 (4%) fecal samples of *C. h. hispidus* collected from seven counties in Texas.

Site of infection: Unknown, oocysts collected from feces.

Material deposited: Phototypes of oocysts in the USNMPC No. 80934. Host skin and skeleton in the ASUMZ, No. 18031 (adult male), October 10, 1987.

Etymology: The species name is derived from *ang* (Gr., vessel), *muri* (L., mouse), and *ensis* (L., belonging to), indicating that this parasite is from a pocket (vessel) mouse.

Remarks: Cyclosporans were described first from a myriapod, *Glomeris* sp., by Schneider (1881), but records from reptiles and mammals, especially insectivores (Pellerdy, 1974), are not uncommon. To date, eight mammalian cyclosporans have been described from moles. The form described here differs from the other *Cyclospora* species by having an oocyst residuum and by the shape and L:W ratio of its sporocysts (1.3 vs 1.6 or larger).

1.4.15 *Cyclospora cayetanensis* (Ortega, 1994)

Description: Oocysts spheroidal, 8.6±0.6 μm (7.7–9.9 μm) with a bilayered wall, 113 nm thickness; outer layer 63 nm and rough; inner layer 50 nm and smooth. A polar body and oocyst residuum are also present. Sporocysts ($n=30$) ovoidal, 4.0 μm wide ±0.4 (3.3–4.4 μm)×6.34 μm long ±0.63 (5.5–7.1 μm). Sporocyst has Stieda and substieda bodies. Sporocyst residuum has large spherical globules. A micropyle was not observed. Sporozoites are 1.2 μm wide vs 9.0 μm long (1.06–1.34 vs 8.0–10.0 μm). The oocyst resembles those of the coccidian genus *Cyclospora* because excystation of the mature oocyst yields two sporocysts, each with two sporozoites.

Taxonomic summary

Synonym: CLB, cyanobacterium-like body, coccidian-like body, blue-green algae.

Type host: *Homo sapiens.*

Type locality: San Juan de Miraflores, a shantytown ~15 km south of Lima, Peru.

Prevalence: 6% (15/230) and 18% (26/147) from two separate prospective cohort studies in children ranging in age from birth to 2.5 years.

Site of infection: Suspected to parasitize jejunum epithelial cells (Bendall et al., 1993). Oocysts recovered from feces.

Sporulation: Exogenous.

Life cycle: Unknown.

Material deposited: Phototypes of oocysts in the USNM Parasite Collection **Accession number:** 83416 document #79; vial (M1461F).

Etymology: The species name combines the name of the university where the principal studies on this parasite were conducted *cayetan* (Cayetano Heredia University, Lima, Peru) and *ensis* (L., belonging to).

Remarks Oocysts stain variably using acid-fast staining techniques. Oocysts autofluoresce green under UV epifluorescence microscopy using a 450–490 DM exciter filter. Although the oocyst is similar to other *Cyclospora* sp. described from insectivores, reptiles, and rodents, it is smaller in size. Ashford (1979) first reported *C. cayetanensis* from humans in New Guinea with characteristics similar to those described previously, but thought it might belong to the genus *Isospora* spp. Individuals presenting with diarrhea and cyanobacterium-like bodies (CLBs) in their stools had jejunal biopsy specimens taken. Intraepithelial coccidia zoites were seen by electron microscopy. Sporulation, but not excystation of CLBs recovered from fecal samples, was attempted. The exact identity of the organism was not determined (Bendall et al., 1993). Until now, *C. cayetanensis* is the only documented *Cyclospora* species known to infect humans (Ortega and Sanchez, 2010; Li et al., 2020). The species caused large foodborne outbreaks of cyclosporiasis in the developed countries in the past decades posing a great deal of public health concern (Li et al., 2020).

1.4.16 *Cyclospora cercopitheci* (Eberhard, 1999)

Description: Ocysts spherical; 8.0–10.0 μm (mean 9.2 μm) in diameter. Outer wall smooth. Wall autofluorescences in UV wavelength.

Type host: *C. aethiops* Linnaeus, 1758, African green or vervet monkey.

Type locality: Gimbie, Wollega Province, Ethiopia.

Prevalence: Found in 6% of the green monkeys sampled.

Site of infection: Unknown, oocysts collected from feces.

Material deposited: Phototypes and syntypes in the US National Parasite Collection, accession number 088837.

Etymology: The species name is derived from the genus name for the primate host from which this parasite was recovered.

Named by: Eberhard et al. in 1999.

Remarks: Sequencing of SSU-rRNA coding region of *C. cercopitheci* from a single African green monkey specimen revealed that there was a heterozygotic position, T or A at position 280. Thus, SSU-rRNA sequences for the two isolates were submitted separately to GenBank and were assigned under the accession numbers AF111184 and AF111185.

1.4.17 *Cyclospora colobi* (Eberhard, 1999)

Description: Oocysts small, spherical, 8.0–9.0 µm (mean 8.3 µm) in diameter. Outer wall smooth. Wall autofluoresces in UV wavelength.

Type host: *C.s guereza* (Ruppell, 1835), colobus monkey.

Type locality: Gimbie, Wollega Province, Ethiopia.

Prevalence: Found in up to 60% of the colobus monkeys sampled.

Site of infection: Unknown, oocysts collected from feces.

Material deposited: Phototypes and syntypes in the US National Parasite Collection, accession number 088838. Sequence of the SSU-rRNA coding region for this species was deposited in GenBank and was assigned under the accession number AF111186.

Etymology: The species name is derived from the genus name of the primate host from which this parasite was recovered.

Named by: Eberhard et al. in 1999.

Remarks: This species is marginally smaller than the two other species described from monkeys, but the overlap in sizes between the species does not allow a clear distinction on the basis of size. Sporulation of material collected from colobus monkeys was poor in comparison with *C. papionis* from baboons, despite the fact that material was collected and handled in a similar fashion.

1.4.18 *Cyclospora papionis* (Eberhard, 1999)

Description: Oocysts spherical, 8–10 µm (mean 8.8 µm) in diameter. Outer wall smooth. Wall autofluoresces in UV wavelength.

Type host: *P. anubis* (Lesson, 1827), olive baboon.
Type locality: Gimbie, Wollega Province, Ethiopia.
Prevalence: Found in >50% of the baboons sampled.
Site of infection: Unknown, oocysts collected from feces.
Material deposited: Phototypes and syntypes in the US National Parasite Collection, accession number 088839. Sequence of the SSU-rRNA coding region for this species was deposited in GenBank and was assigned under the accession number AF111187.
Etymology: The species name is derived from the genus name for the primate host from which this parasite was recovered.
Named by: Eberhard et al. in 1999.
Remarks: More than 90% of the oocysts collected from baboons underwent sporulation in virtually all of the positive samples.

1.4.19 *Cyclospora schneideri* (Lainson, 2005)

Description: Mature oocysts ovoid to subspherical or, more rarely, spherical, $15.1–25.7 \times 13.8–20.1\,\mu m$ (mean $19.8 \times 16.6\,\mu m$), shape index 1–1.3 (mean 1.2) ($n=100$). No oocyst residuum or polar bodies present. Oocyst wall approximately 0.5–1 thick, colorless, smooth, and apparently of a single layer: no micropyle or striations. It is fragile and soon becomes highly deformed. The two dizoic sporocysts average $11.3 \times 8.3–15.1 \times 9.9\,\mu m$ (mean $13.6 \times 9.4\,\mu m$), shape index 1.2–1.5 (mean 1.4) ($n=77$): there is an inconspicuous nipple-like Stieda body. The sporozoites measure $11–13.0 \times 2.5–3\,\mu m$ ($n=13$), and curve slightly around a sporocystic residuum of fine granules and larger globules. Refractile bodies were not detected.

Endogenous stages: The parasites develop, in conspicuous parasitophorous vacuoles, in the cytoplasm of the epithelial cells of the small intestine. In histological sections of the infected gut, most of the developing parasites were clearly located above the host cell nucleus, but it is possible that others commenced development below and, with growth, eventually positioned themselves between or above the nuclei. Mature meronts were scanty but appeared to be of a single, small in size of approximately $16 \times 14\,\mu m$ ($n=4$): they produce 6–12 merozoites, measuring an average of $10 \times 2.5\,\mu m$ ($n=4$) and segmentation leaves no residuum. Growing microgamonts reach up to $33 \times 26\,\mu m$ and contain many bulky, heavily stained nuclei distributed predominantly at the periphery of the parasite. Mature forms have a residuum containing a few big vacuoles, and shed a large number of microgametes measuring approximately $5.0 \times 1\,\mu m$. Young macrogamonts have a poorly staining nucleus containing a densely staining karyosome. Mature forms may reach up to $24 \times 20\,\mu m$ $(15 \times 10–24 \times 20\,\mu m)$ $(n = 10)$ and contain very prominent small and large wall-forming bodies. The wide size range of the mature macrogamonts results in an equally wide range in the size of the zygotes and the oocysts.

Sporulation: Exogenous, in approximately 1 week.

Type host: The snake *Anilius scytale scytale* (Linnaeus), (Aniliidae).

Type locality: Capanema, state of Pará, North Brazil.

Type material: Oocysts in 10% buffered formalin, histological sections of the endogenous stages and phototypes in the Department of Parasitology, Instituto Evandro Chagas and the Muséum National d'Histoire Naturelle, Paris: Accession No. 2257.

Prevalence: Uncertain. Only two *Anilius scytale scytale* (Aniliidae) were examined and both were infected.

Pathology: No apparent pathology.

Etymology: The specific name is in honor of Aimé Schneider, who found the genus *Cyclospora*.

Named by: Lainson in 2005.

1.4.20 *Cyclospora macacae* (Li, 2015)

Description: Oocysts measure $8.49 \pm 0.55 \times 8.49 \pm 0.49\,\mu m$ with a length/width shape index of 1.02 $(n = 11)$. Two sporocysts are seen in each oocyst.

Type host: Rhesus monkeys (*M. mulatta*).

Other natural hosts: Crab-eating macaques (*M. fascicularis*).

Type locality: Guiyang, Guizhou Province, China.

Prevalence: Found in 6.6% of the rhesus monkeys sampled.

Site of infection: Unknown, oocysts collected from feces.

Material deposited: The SSU rRNA sequence of this species has been deposited in GenBank under the accession number KP335196.

Etymology: The species name *C. macacae* is derived from the genus name of its host (*M. mulatta*) from which this parasite was recovered.

Named by: Li N et al. in 2015.

Remarks: Based on the unique genetic feature and apparent restriction to the macaque monkeys, the newly identified *Cyclospora* parasite was named as *C. macacae* n. sp.

1.4.21 *Cyclospora duszynskii* (McAllister et al., 2018)

Description: Oocyst $(n = 90)$ subspheroidal, $10.0–12.0 \times 9.0–11.0\,\mu m$ (mean $11.4 \times 10.0\,\mu m$); L:W ratio 1.0–1.2 (mean 1.1); wall smooth, thin, bi-layered, *c.* 0.7, inner layer *c.* 0.2, light brown outer layer *c.*0.5. Micropyle and oocyst residuum absent, single polar granule present. Sporocysts ($n = 175$) two, ellipsoidal, $6.0–10.0 \times 4.0–7.0\,\mu m$ (mean $7.2 \times 5.4\,\mu m$); L:W ratio 1.0– 1.6 (mean 1.3); wall smooth, thin and unilayered, light brown, c. 0.2 thick. Indistinct Stieda body present, sub-Stieda and para-Stieda bodies absent; sporocyst residuum medium to large granules of different sizes along the edge of sporocyst. Sporozoites (two, not measured) banana–shaped, with a spheroidal anterior and posterior refractile bodies; nucleus difficult to discern.

Type host: *S. aquaticus* (Linnaeus, 1758) (Mammalia, Soricomorpha, Talpidae), eastern mole; adult (not measured).

Type locality: Bentonville (36°21′58.2186″W, 94°14′38.634″W), Benton County, Arkansas, USA.

Other locality: El Dorado (33°13′0.5298″N, 92°35′9.7548″W), Union County, Arkansas, USA (two adult *S. aquaticus* (118 and 157 mm in total length) collected on 2013).

Type material: Photosyntypes of sporulated oocysts are deposited as HWML 139341.

Prevalence: Found in 3 of the 7 (43%) samples tested—overall; in 1 of the 3 (33%) samples tested in Benton County, Arkansas, USA; in 2 of the 3 (50%) samples tested in Union County, Arkansas, USA.

Sporulation time: Unknown; oocysts were sporulated when examined.

Site of infect ion: Unknown; oocysts recovered from feces.

ZooBank registration: To comply with the regulations set out in article 8.5 of the amended 2012 version of the International Code of Zoological Nomenclature (ICZN, 2012), details of the new species have been submitted to ZooBank. The Life Science Identifier (LSID) for *Cyclospora duszynskii*. sp. is urn:lsid:zoobank.org:act:67ED7C1C-A8FC-449B-9D06-6066DB425264.

Etymology: The specific epithet is given in honor of Dr. Donald W. Duszynski (Emeritus Professor of Biology, University of New Mexico, Albuquerque, New Mexico, USA), Dean of American coccidiologists, for his many works on the coccidia of vertebrates, including moles.

Named by: McAllister et al. in 2018.

Remarks: This new species is comparable only to cyclosporan species from North American moles of the family Talpidae Fischer. None of the five *Cyclospora* spp. (*C. ashtabulensis*, *C. duszynskii*, *C. megacephali*, *C. parascalopi*, *C. yatesi*) from moles possess oocysts as minute as the new species. There is a previously described species from *S. aquaticus* (hosts from Texas, USA), the oocysts of *C. megacephali* (Ford and Duszynski, 1988) is similar, but the subspheroidal oocysts are large and measure $18.9 \times 15.7\,\mu m$

(L:W ratio = 1.2), the sporocysts are large, 15.0 × 7.2 μm (L:W of 2.1), and there is a large cap-like Stieda body. Oocysts of *C. ashtabulensis* Ford & Duszynski, 1989 from hairy-tailed mole, *P. breweri* (Bachman), from Ohio, USA are also large and measure 18.0 × 14.3 μm and also do not possess a polar granule which is present in the new species. *C. parascalopi* Ford & Duszynski, 1989 from *P. breweri* from Massachusetts and Ohio has large oocysts measuring 16.5 × 13.6 μm (L:W = 1.2), without a polar granule. Both these latter species from *P. breweri* also have a prominent cap-like Stieda body which is not present in the new species (Ford and Duszynski, 1988, 1989). There are also two species of *Cyclospora* from European moles, *T. europaea* Linnaeus, i.e., *C. caryolytica* Schaudinn, 1902 from Bulgaria, Germany and Italy, and *C. talpae* Pellérdy & Tanyi, 1968 from Austria, Bulgaria, England, and Hungary. However, neither of these taxa is similar to the new species and, more importantly, they are also widely separated geographically from hosts in the Western Hemisphere. Based on the differences in morphological and morphometric characteristics noted above, *C. duszynskii* is considered a species new to science. Moreover, to date, it is the smallest cyclosporan reported from moles as well as the first species from a mole in Arkansas and the second species known from *S. aquaticus*.

1.4.22 *Cyclospora yatesi* (McAllister et al., 2018)

Description: Oocysts ($n = 53$) are subspheroidal to ovoidal, 12.0–18.0 × 10.0–17.0 μm (mean 17.0 × 15.2 μm); L:W ratio 1.0–1.2 (mean 1.1). Wall ornate, bilayered, c. 1.3 thick, inner layer c. 0.7, yellowish-brown outer layer c. 0.6. Micropyle and oocyst residuum absent, single polar granule present. Sporocysts ($n = 106$) two, ellipsoidal 6.0–12.0 × 5.0–10.0 (mean 9.7 × 7.3); L:W ratio 0.7–1.9 (mean 1.3); wall smooth, unilayered, colorless, c. 0.2 thick. Indistinct Stieda body present, sub-Stieda and para-Stieda bodies absent; sporocyst residuum medium to large granules of different sizes along the edge of sporocyst. Sporozoites (two, not measured) banana-shaped, with a spheroidal anterior and posterior refractile bodies; nucleus difficult to discern.

    Type host: *S. aquaticus* (Linnaeus, 1758) (Mammalia, Soricomorpha, Talpidae), eastern mole; adult collected.

    Type locality: El Dorado (33°13′0.5298″N, 92°35′9.7548″W), Union County, Arkansas, USA.

    Other locality: Bentonville (36°21′58.2186″W, 94°14′38.634″W), Benton County, Arkansas, USA [1 adult (not measured) collected 26.x.2016].

Type material: Photosyntypes of sporulated oocysts are deposited as HWML 139342.

Prevalence: Found in 3 of the 7 (43%) fecal samples—overall; in 1 of the 3 (33%) samples in Benton County, Arkansas, USA; in 2 of the 3 (67%) samples in Union County, Arkansas, USA.

Sporulation time: Unknown; oocysts were sporulated when examined.

Site of infect ion: Unknown; oocysts recovered from feces.

ZooBank registration: To comply with the regulations set out in article 8.5 of the amended 2012 version of the International Code of Zoological Nomenclature (ICZN, 2012), details of the new species have been submitted to ZooBank. The Life Science Identifier (LSID) for *C. yatesi* n. sp. is urn:lsid: zoobank.org: act: 6F9B0451-E018-4F87-8C6E-7F026BF4A0DD.

Etymology: The specific epithet is given in honor of the late Dr. Terry L. Yates (1950–2007) (University of New Mexico, Albuquerque, New Mexico, USA), renowned mammalogist and mole expert who is credited with discovering the source of the hantavirus in the American Southwest in 1993.

Named by: McAllister et al. in 2018.

Remarks: The new taxon is comparable only to the cyclosporan species from North American moles of the family Talpidae. The species possesses oocysts with sculptured outer walls that are similar in size and wall morphology to two previously described cyclosporans from *P. breweri*. Both *C. ashtabulensis* and *C. parascalopi* have sculptured outer walls on their oocysts and also have very different sporocysts with crescent-shaped caps or thick cap-like coverings on their Stieda bodies that the new species does not possess. The only cyclosporan from *S. aquaticus*, *C. megacephali* has a smooth outer wall on its oocysts. Based on the differences in morphological and morphometric characteristics noted above, *C. yatesi* is considered a species new to science. It also represents the third cyclosporan from *S. aquaticus* as well as another species from an Arkansas mole.

1.4.23 Some unnamed *Cyclospora*-like organisms in animals

Several other *Cyclospora* species or *Cyclospora*-like organisms have been reported in various animals (Table 1.2), including five *Cyclospora* species in nonhuman primates (Eberhard et al., 1999, 2001; Ortega and Sanchez, 2010; Li et al., 2015). Among the animals, *Cyclospora*-like organisms have been described in dogs, cattle, chickens, rats/house mice, birds, monkeys, shellfish, etc. (Sherchand and Cross, 2001; Chu et al., 2004; Li et al., 2007;

Table 1.2 Reports of *Cyclospora* spp. or *Cyclospora*-like organisms among animals.

Host type	Host common name	Country (site)	Detection method	Sample number	Positive number	Infection rate (%)
Nonhuman primate	Golden snub-nosed monkey	China, Shaanxi	PCR	71	2	2.8
	Crab-eating macaque	China, Guangxi	PCR	205	1	0.5
	Rhesus macaque	China, Guizhou	PCR	411	28	6.8
	Monkey	China	Light microscopy	3349	7	0.2
	Bioko drill (*Mandrillus leucophaeus poensis*)	Equatorial Guinea	PCR	51	11	21.6
	Vervet monkey	Ethiopia	Modified Ziehl-Neelsen satin	41	9	22.0
	Monkey	Italy	qPCR	119	11	9.2
	Nonhuman primates	Kenya	PCR	511	81	1.6
	Monkey	Nepal	PCR	3	1	33.3
	Nonhuman primates	Spain	Modified Ziehl-Neelsen satin	18	6	33.3
	Howler monkey	US		96	17	17.7
	Baboon	Ethiopia	Modified Ziehl-Neelsen satin	59	8	13.6
	Baboon	Kenya	PCR	235	42	17.9
	Baboon	Tanzania	PCR		3 cases	
Carnivore	Dog	Brazil, São Paulo	–		2 cases	
	Dog	Egypt	Light microscopy	130	1	0.8
	Dog	Nepal	–	90	2	2.2
	Dog	Nepal	PCR	14	2	14.3
	Carnivorous animals	Spain	Modified Ziehl-Neelsen satin	72	3	4.2

Category	Host	Location	Method	Sample	Cases	%
Artiodactyla	Dairy cattle	China, Guangzhou	PCR–RFLP		2 cases	
	Dairy cattle	China	PCR–OLA	168	6	3.6
	Claves	Japan	PCR		3 cases	
	Artiodactyla animals	Spain	Modified Ziehl–Neelsen satin	198	18	9.1
Aves	Chicken	Mexico	Kinyoun's acid-fast stain; autofluorescence under UV			Cases
	Chicken	Nepal	–	110	3	2.7
	Large-billed crow	Malaysia	Modified Ziehl–Neelsen satin	106	6	5.7
	Chicken	Nepal	PCR	3	1	33.3
	Birds	Spain	Harada–Mori technique satin	984	23	2.3
Others	Rat/house mice	Nepal	–	50	2	4.0
	Cockroach	Thailand, Samutprakarm	Modified acid fast stain	920	10	1.3
	Wild shellfish	Tunisia	qPCR	1255	526	41.9
	Edible shellfish	Turkey (Bays of Izmir and Mersin)	qPCR and HRM	53	14	26.4

HRM: high-resolution melting analysis.

Cordón et al., 2008; Aksoy et al., 2014; Helenbrook et al., 2015). They are also observed in environmental samples (Ghozzi et al., 2017). The Asian freshwater clams (*Corbicula fluminea*) can recover oocysts of *C. cayetanensis* by artificial infection contamination, thus could be used as a biological indicator of water contamination with oocysts (Graczyk et al., 1998). In one study in Nepal, the households keeping livestock had higher *Cyclospora* infection rates (Bhandari et al., 2015).

1.5 Life cycle of *Cyclospora*

The life cycle of human infectious *C. cayetanensis* is well described, where the infection occurs mainly via fecal-oral transmission route. Fresh (un-sporulated) oocysts are excreted in stool. Oocysts are spheroid, 8–10 μm in diameter, and contain indistinguishable protoplasm (Brown and Rotschafer, 1999). In the environment outside of the host, the freshly excreted oocysts are not infectious until complete sporulation, which occurs within a few days to weeks at the maximum in temperatures between 22°C and 30°C. Storage at either 4°C or 37°C retards sporulation (Smith et al., 1997). The sporulation of the oocysts occurs irrespective of whether they are stored in deionized water or in potassium dichromate solution, which results in the division of the sporont into two sporocysts, each containing two elongated sporozoites (Smith et al., 1997). During this time, food or water can serve as a vehicle for *Cyclospora* transmission. Once the sporulated oocysts in food, water, or soil are ingested by a new host, the mature oocysts usually excyst in the small bowel, with sporozoites being released to invade epithelial cells of the upper small intestine (duodenum or jejunum) (Ortega and Sanchez, 2010).

The presence of both asexual and sexual stages in the same host suggests that the life cycle of the microorganism can be completed within one host (Ortega et al., 1997). Intracellular development stages begin with the formation of intracytoplasmic parasitophorous vacuoles in intestinal epithelium cells (Sun et al., 1996; Ortega and Sanchez, 2010), which are sometimes also observed in biliary epithelium cells (Zar et al., 2001). Asexual multiplication results in type I and II meronts (Ortega et al., 1997). Type I meronts give rise to 8–12 merozoites that then infect neighboring epithelial cells; this type of asexual reproduction is often quite prolific. Type II meronts form later, releasing four merozoites to invade neighboring cells. Some of these meronts form macrogametes whereas others undergo multiple fission events to form microgametocytes containing flagellated microgametes (Ortega et al., 1997).

The macrogametocyte is fertilized by the microgametocyte and produces a zygote in the sexual stage. Once fertilization occurs, an environmentally resistant wall is formed, and the oocyst is excreted from the host into the environment as unsporulated oocysts in the feces (Shields and Olson, 2003; Ortega and Sanchez, 2010).

Besides *C. cayetanensis*, the life cycles of some other *Cyclospora* species in animals are described. Schaudinn described the asexual and sexual stages of *C. caryolytica* in both the small and the large intestine of the mole, where they develop within the nucleus of the epithelial cells. With the growth of these stages, the nucleus disintegrates and the host cell becomes a mere sac containing the parasite: a heavy infection may result in fatal enteritis. Schaudinn noted two types of meronts and suggested that the one producing larger merozoites gave rise to the macrogamonts, while the other gave smaller merozoites which were destined to become microgamonts (Lainson, 2005). Tanabe (1938) was unable to demonstrate more than a single type of meront for what he considered to be *C. caryolytica* in *M. wogura coreana* and suggested that Schaudinn was dealing with a mixed infection of that parasite and the merogonic stages of a concomitant Eimeria infection. The consensus of opinion now is that such morphologically different asexual stages merely represent different generations of meronts rather than a sexual dimorphism: Lainson (1965), for example, noted three different types of merozoites produced during the asexual division of *C. niniae* in the snake *Ninia sebae sebae*. In typical eimeriid fashion, the microgamont of *C. caryolitica* produces a large number of flagellated microgametes and, following fertilization of the macrogamonts and development of a resistant membrane around the zygote, the resulting oocysts are expelled, unsporulated, in the feces. Sporulation is completed in 4–5 days, with the formation of two sporocysts, each containing two sporozoites and a sporocystic residuum (Lainson, 2005). Subsequently, however, Pellérdy and Tanyi (1968) described the oocysts of a species in the European mole and named it *C. talpae*. They found microgamonts and macrogamonts in the liver and later in 1990, Mohamed and Molyneux (1990) showed that these sexual stages developed within the nucleus of the bile-duct epithelial cells. Merogony appears to be limited to mononuclear cells in the capillary sinusoids of the liver. Oocysts entering the intestine with the bile are voided in the feces and exogenous sporulation is completed in about 2 weeks. In more recent years, a detailed description of the life cycle stages of *C. cayetanensis* reported in a 33-year-old male with human immunodeficiency virus facilitated histopathologic diagnosis of this parasite (Dubey et al., 2020). It was shown that the parasite's development more closely resembles that of *Cystoisospora* than *Eimeria* and that the parasite has multiple nuclei per immature meront indicating schizogony, and we have undermined evidence for a Type II meront (Dubey et al., 2020).

1.6 Conclusion

With the large number of human cyclosporiasis outbreaks in North America, enormous studies on different issues of *Cyclospora*, such as biology, epidemiology, outbreak investigation, infection source tracking, detection technique, treatment, and prevention have been conducted across the world. The studies have resulted in 22 valid species of *Cyclospora* and some *Cyclospora*-like unnamed organisms in many animal and human hosts. Taxonomically, the genus *Cyclospora* belongs to family Eimeriidae under the subclass Coccidiasina and subphylum Apicomplexa. The biology and morphology studies documented that the oocysts of *Cyclospora* parasite differ in forms by different species under light microscopy, and the most commonly reported forms are spheroidal, subspheroidal, ovoid, or ellipsoidal. Oocysts of some species, such as *C. glomericola*, *C. schneider*, *C. angimurinensis*, are large, while oocysts of others, such as *C. cayetanensis*, *C. colobi*, *C. papionis*, *C. macacae*, are small. In general, the oocyst wall of *Cyclospora* autofluorescences under fluorescence microscopy, which is an important characteristic of this parasite. Attempts have been made to study the life cycle of *Cyclospora* spp. on many occasions and a convincing description was obtained only for human infections of *C. cayetanensis* that mainly transmited via fecal-oral route. The parasite completes both asexual (sporulation) and sexual (gametogamy) stages in its life cycle, even in the same host, indicating the one host life cycle of the parasite.

References

Abanyie, F., Harvey, R.R., Harris, J.R., Wiegand, R.E., Gaul, L., Desvignes-Kendrick, M., Irvin, K., Williams, I., Hall, R.L., Herwaldt, B., Gray, E.B., Qvarnstrom, Y., Wise, M.E., Cantu, V., Cantey, P.T., Bosch, S., DA Silva, A.J., Fields, A., Bishop, H., Wellman, A., Beal, J., Wilson, N., Fiore, A.E., Tauxe, R., Lance, S., Slutsker, L., Parise, M., Multistate cyclosporiasis outbreak investigation team, 2015. 2013 multistate outbreaks of *Cyclospora cayetanensis* infections associated with fresh produce: focus on the Texas investigations. Epidemiol. Infect. 143, 3451–3458.
Aksoy, U., Marangi, M., Papini, R., Ozkoc, S., Bayram Delibas, S., Giangaspero, A., 2014. Detection of *Toxoplasma gondii* and *Cyclospora cayetanensis* in *Mytilus galloprovincialis* from Izmir Province coast (Turkey) by real time PCR/high-resolution melting analysis (HRM). Food Microbiol. 44, 128–135.

Almeria, S., Cinar, H.N., Dubey, J.P., 2019. *Cyclospora cayetanensis* and cyclosporiasis: an update. Microorganisms 7, 317.

Ashford, R.W., 1979. Occurrence of an undescribed coccidian in man in Papua New Guinea. Ann. Trop. Med. Parasitol. 73, 497–500.

Ashford, R.W., Warhurst, D.C., Reid, G.D.F., 1993. Human infection with cyanobacterium-like bodies. Lancet 341, 1034.

Bhandari, D., Tandukar, S., Parajuli, H., Thapa, P., Chaudhary, P., Shrestha, D., Shah, P.K., Sherchan, J.B., Sherchand, J.B., 2015. *Cyclospora* infection among school children in Kathmandu, Nepal: prevalence and associated risk factors. Trop. Med. Health 43, 211–216.

Brown, G.H., Rotschafer, J.C., 1999. *Cyclospora*: review of an emerging parasite. Pharmacotherapy 19, 70–75.

Casillas, S.M., Bennett, C., Straily, A., 2018. Notes from the field: multiple cyclosporiasis outbreaks - United States, 2018. MMWR Morb. Mortal. Wkly Rep. 67, 1101–1102.

Chu, D.M., Sherchand, J.B., Cross, J.H., Orlandi, P.A., 2004. Detection of *Cyclospora cayetanensis* in animal fecal isolates from Nepal using an FTA filter-base polymerase chain reaction method. Am. J. Trop. Med. Hyg. 71, 373–379.

Clarke, S.C., McIntyre, M., 1996. Modified detergent Ziehl-Neelsen technique for the staining of *Cyclospora cayetanensis*. J. Clin. Pathol. 49, 511–512.

Cordón, G.P., Prados, A.H., Romero, D., Moreno, M.S., Pontes, A., Osuna, A., Rosales, M.J., 2008. Intestinal parasitism in the animals of the zoological garden "Peña Escrita" (Almuñecar, Spain). Vet. Parasitol. 156, 302–309.

Dubey, J.P., Almeria, S., Mowery, J., Fortes, J., 2020. Endogenous developmental cycle of the human coccidian *Cyclospora cayetanensis*. J. Parasitol. 106, 295–307.

Duszynski, D.W., Wattam, A.R., 1988. Coccidian parasites (Apicomplexa: Eimeriidae) from insectivores IV. Four new species in *Talpa europaea* from England. J. Protozool. 35, 58–62.

Eberhard, M.L., da Silva, A.J., Lilley, B.G., Pieniazek, N.J., 1999. Morphologic and molecular characterization of new *Cyclospora* species from Ethiopian monkeys: *C. cercopitheci* sp.n., *C. colobi* sp.n., and *C. papionis* sp.n. Emerg. Infect. Dis. 5, 651–658.

Eberhard, M.L., Njenga, M.N., DaSilva, A.J., Owino, D., Nace, E.K., Won, K.Y., Mwenda, J.M., 2001. A survey for *Cyclospora* spp. in Kenyan primates, with some notes on its biology. J. Parasitol. 87, 1394–1397.

Ford, P.L., Duszynski, D.W., 1988. Coccidian parasites from insectivores VI. Six new species from the Eastern mole *Scalopus aquaticus*. J. Protozool. 35, 223–226.

Ford, P.L., Duszynski, D.W., McAllister, C.T., 1990. Coccidia (Apicomplexa) from heteromyid rodents in the Southwestern United States, Baja California, and Northern Mexico, with three new species from *Chaetodipus hispidus*. J. Parasitol. 76, 325–333.

Ghozzi, K., Marangi, M., Papini, R., Lahmar, I., Challouf, R., Houas, N., Ben Dhiab, R., Normanno, G., Babba, H., Giangaspero, A., 2017. First report of Tunisian coastal water contamination by protozoan parasites using mollusk bivalves as biological indicators. Mar. Pollut. Bull. 117, 197–202.

Graczyk, T.K., Ortega, Y.R., Conn, D.B., 1998. Recovery of waterborne oocysts of *Cyclospora cayetanensis* by Asian freshwater clams (*Corbicula fluminea*). Am. J. Trop. Med. Hyg. 59, 928–932.

Helenbrook, W.D., Wade, S.E., Shields, W.M., Stehman, S.V., Whipps, C.M., 2015. Gastrointestinal parasites of ecuadorian mantled howler monkeys (*Alouatta palliata aequatorialis*) based on fecal analysis. J. Parasitol. 101, 341–350.

Herwaldt, B.L., 2000. *Cyclospora cayetanensis*: a review, focusing on the outbreaks of cyclosporiasis in the 1990s. Clin. Infect. Dis. 31, 1040–1057.

Herwaldt, B.L., Ackers, M.L., 1997. An outbreak in 1996 of cyclosporiasis associated with imported raspberries. The *Cyclospora* working group. N. Engl. J. Med. 336, 1548–1556.

Huang, P., Weber, J.T., Sosin, D.M., Griffin, P.M., Long, E.G., Murphy, J.J., Kocka, F., Peters, C., Kallick, C., 1995. The first reported outbreak of diarrheal illness associated with *Cyclospora* in the United States. Ann. Intern. Med. 123, 409–414.

Lainson, R., 1965. Parasitological studies in British Honduras II. *Cyclospora niniae* sp.n. (Eimeriidae: Cyclosporinae) from the snake *Ninia sebae sebae* (Colubridae). Ann. Trop. Med. Parasitol. 59, 159–163.

Lainson, R., 2005. The genus *Cyclospora* (Apicomplexa: Eimeriidae), with a description of *Cyclospora schneideri* n.sp. in the snake *Anilius scytale scytale* (Aniliidae) from Amazonian Brazil-a review. Mem. Inst. Oswaldo Cruz 100, 103–110.

Li, G., Xiao, S., Zhou, R., Li, W., Wadeh, H., 2007. Molecular characterization of *Cyclospora*-like organism from dairy cattle. Parasitol. Res. 100, 955–961.

Li, N., Ye, J., Arrowood, M.J., Ma, J., Wang, L., Xu, H., Feng, Y., Xiao, L., 2015. Identification and morphologic and molecular characterization of *Cyclospora macacae* n. sp. from rhesus monkeys in China. Parasitol. Res. 114, 1811–1816.

Li, J., Wang, R., Chen, Y., Xiao, L., Zhang, L., 2020. *Cyclospora cayetanensis* infection in humans: biological characteristics, clinical features, epidemiology, detection method, and treatment. Parasitology 147, 160–170.

Liu, S., Wang, L., Zheng, H., Xu, Z., Roellig, D.M., Li, N., Frace, M.A., Tang, K., Arrowood, M.J., Moss, D.M., Zhang, L., Feng, Y., Xiao, L., 2016. Comparative genomics reveals *Cyclospora cayetanensis* possesses coccidia-like metabolism and invasion components but unique surface antigens. BMC Genomics 17, 316.

Long, E.G., White, E.H., Carmichael, W.W., Quinlisk, P.M., Raja, R., Swisher, B.L., Daugharty, H., Cohen, M.T., 1991. Morphological and staining characteristics of a cyanobacterium-like organism associated with diarrhea. J. Infect. Dis. 164, 199–202.

McAllister, C.T., Motriuk-Smith, D., Kerr, C.M., 2018. Three new coccidians (*Cyclospora*, *Eimeria*) from eastern moles, *Scalopus aquaticus* (Linnaeus) (Mammalia: Soricomorpha: Talpidae) from Arkansas, USA. Syst. Parasitol. 95, 271–279.

Ortega, Y.R., Sanchez, R., 2010. Update on *Cyclospora cayetanensis*, a food-borne and waterborne parasite. Clin. Microbiol. Rev. 23, 218–234.

Mohamed, H.A., Molyneux, D.H., 1990. Developmental stages of *Cyclospora talpae* in the liver and bile duct of the mole *Talpa europaea*. Parasitology 101, 345–350.

Ortega, Y.R., Gilman, R.H., Sterling, C.R., 1994. A new coccidian parasite (Apicomplexa: Eimeriidae) from humans. J. Parasitol. 80, 625–629.

Ortega, Y.R., Nagle, R., Gilman, R.H., Watanabe, J., Miyagui, J., Quispe, H., Kanagusuku, P., Roxas, C., Sterling, C.R., 1997. Pathologic and clinical findings in patients with cyclosporiasis and a description of intracellular parasite life-cycle stages. J. Infect. Dis. 176, 1584–1589.

Pellérdy, L., Tanyi, Z., 1968. *Cyclospora talpae* sp.n. (Protozoa: Sporozoa) from the liver of *Talpa europaea*. Folia Parasitol. (Praha). 15, 275–277.

Relman, D.A., Schmidt, T.M., Gajadhar, A., Sogin, M., Cross, J., Yoder, K., Sethabutr, O., Echeverria, P., 1996. Molecular phylogenetic analysis of *Cyclospora*, the human intestinal pathogen, suggests that it is closely related to *Eimeria* species. J. Infect. Dis. 173, 440–445.

Sherchand, J.B., Cross, J.H., 2001. Emerging pathogen *Cyclospora cayetanensis* infection in Nepal. Southeast Asian J. Trop. Med. Public Health 32, 143–150.

Shields, J.M., Olson, B.H., 2003. *Cyclospora cayetanensis*: a review of an emerging parasitic coccidian. Int. J. Parasitol. 33, 371–391.

Smith, H.V., Paton, C.A., Mitambo, M.M., Girdwood, R.W., 1997. Sporulation of *Cyclospora* sp. oocysts. Appl. Environ. Microbiol. 63, 1631–1632.

Sun, T., Ilardi, C.F., Asnis, D., Bresciani, A.R., Goldenberg, S., Roberts, B., Teichberg, S., 1996. Light and electron microscopic identification of *Cyclospora* species in the small intestine. Evidence of the presence of asexual life cycle in human host. Am. J. Clin. Pathol. 105, 216–220.

Tanabe, M., 1938. On three species of coccidia of the mole, *Mogera wogura coreana* Thomas, with special reference to the life history of *Cyclospora caryolytica*. Keijo J. Med. 9, 21–52.

Zar, F.A., El-Bayoumi, E., Yungbluth, M.M., 2001. Histologic proof of acalculous cholecystitis due to *Cyclospora cayetanensis*. Clin. Infect. Dis. 33, E140–E141.

Zhou, Y., Lv, B., Wang, Q., Wang, R., Jian, F., Zhang, L., Ning, C., Fu, K., Wang, Y., Qi, M., Yao, H., Zhao, J., Zhang, X., Sun, Y., Shi, K., Arrowood, M.J., Xiao, L., 2011. Prevalence and molecular characterization of *Cyclospora cayetanensis*, Henan, China. Emerg. Infect. Dis. 17, 1887–1890.

CHAPTER 2

Molecular characteristics

Contents

2.1 Introduction

Characteristics of polymorphic regions of the *Cyclospora* genome had been studied to better understand the microorganism's mode of infection and molecular epidemiology. Some loci of *Cyclospora* were used to precisely identify and trace the *Cyclospora* infections, such as small subunit ribosomal RNA (SSU rRNA) gene (Sulaiman et al., 2014), internal transcribed spacer (ITS) (Olivier et al., 2001), and 70 kDa heat shock protein (HSP70) locus (Sulaiman et al., 2013).

Up to now, the whole genome of *Cyclospora cayetanensis* is obtained, which includes the mitochondrial genome (Cinar et al., 2015; Ogedengbe et al., 2015; Tang et al., 2015), apicoplast genome (Tang et al., 2015; Liu et al., 2016), and chromosome genome (Liu et al., 2016). Tracing the source of infection is facilitated by the genomic comparison of isolates. *Cyclospora* can also be clearly identified and differentiated from other protozoan parasites involved in foodborne or waterborne outbreaks by their genomic differences. These useful genotyping tools could be helpful in initial source-tracking studies and in distinguishing different case clusters, especially during cyclosporiasis outbreaks.

2.2 Molecular characteristics of the main loci

2.2.1 Molecular characteristics of *C. cayetanensis* in human

Small subunit ribosomal RNA (SSU rRNA) gene sequences show minimal genetic diversity among *C. cayetanensis* isolates around the world (Sulaiman et al., 2014), and *C. cayetanensis* is genetically related to members of the *Eimeria* genus in phylogenetic analysis (Relman et al., 1996). However, internal transcribed spacer (ITS) sequences are highly variable within and between samples, and the variability does not correlate with geographic origin of the samples (Olivier et al., 2001). It has been determined that ITS sequence variability exists at individual-genome level in *C. cayetanensis* and approaches or exceeds the variability exhibited among oocysts (Riner et al., 2010). These multiple sequences could represent multiple clones from a single clinical source or, more likely, variability of the ITS region among different copies of the rRNA gene unit (Adam et al., 2000).

No genetic polymorphism was observed in regions of the 70-kDa heat shock proteins (HSP70) locus characterized in previous study (Sulaiman et al., 2013), these results also support a lack of geographic segregation and the existence of a genetically homogeneous population in *C. cayetanensis* parasites at this genetic locus (Sulaiman et al., 2014).

Over the past few decades, several conventional, nested, and quantitative PCR (qPCR) as well as multiplex PCR assays (together with other parasites) are developed for the identification of *Cyclospora* (Relman et al., 1996; Varma et al., 2003; Taniuchi et al., 2011; Almeria et al., 2019; Li et al., 2020). There is one commercially available fully automated system involving high-order multiplex PCR reactions that is capable of detecting *C. cayetanensis* with high sensitivity and specificity (Buss et al., 2015). The multiplex Biofire (Salt Lake City, UT, USA) FilmArray Gastrointestinal Panel is a commercially available DNA-based technology for the detection of *C. cayetanensis* (Ryan et al., 2017; Hitchcock et al., 2019).

Recently, a molecular diagnostic method utilizing multiplex real-time PCR and a T4 phage internal control has been devised for the simultaneous detection of *Cryptosporidium parvum*, *Giardia lamblia*, and *C. cayetanensis* in human stools (Shin et al., 2018). The QIAstat gastrointestinal panel can detect a large range of acute gastroenteritis pathogens with a high sensitivity, including *C. cayetanensis* (Hannet et al., 2019). Molecular-based detection methods have the capacity to screen a number of organisms at a time using multiplex platforms and to detect them rapidly with high sensitivity (even detection of a single oocyst), thus overcoming some of the limitations of

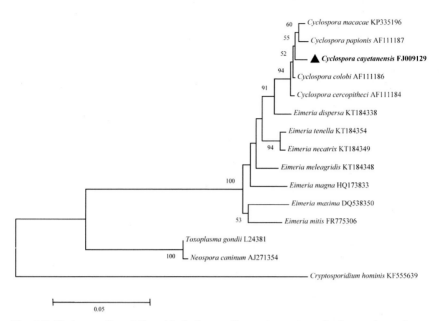

Fig. 2.1 Phylogenetic relationship between *C. cayetanensis* and other apicomplexan protozoa. Phylogeny inferred with a neighbor-joining analysis of small-subunit ribosomal RNA gene sequences (A) reported by Li et al. (2017), based on distances calculated with the Kimura 2-parameter model. Bootstrap values > 50% from 1000 replicates are shown at the nodes. Scale bars indicate estimated substitutions per site.

microscopy-based diagnosis. These molecular methods are widely used in laboratory testing or sample verification in clinic.

Previous studies using 18S rRNA and ITS sequences place *C. cayetanensis* in a clade with chicken eimerids (Fig. 2.1). It constructed a phylogenetic tree using currently available *Eimeria* spp. 18S rRNA gene sequences, and *C. cayetanensis* 18S rRNA gene. In our 18S rRNA bootstrap analysis, *C. cayetanensis* appears to cluster with *Eimeria meleagrimitis*. Mammalian coccidians *Eimeria magna* and *Eimeria bovis* are found to be closely related to each other, but located in a clade different from *C. cayetanensis* tree location.

2.2.2 Molecular characteristics of animals source *Cyclospora*

Only some of the animals originated *Cyclospora* species had molecular data, for example, *Cyclospora cercopitheci* in vervet monkeys (*Cercopithecus aethiops*), *Cyclospora colobi* in colobus monkeys (*Colobus guereza*), and *Cyclospora papionis* in olive baboons (*Papio anubis*) were characterized in 1999 (Eberhard et al., 1999); *Cyclospora macacae* was described in rhesus monkeys (*Macaca mulatta*) in 2015 (Li et al., 2015a, b); and *Cyclospora duszynskii* and *Cyclospora yatesi* were characterized in moles (*Scalopus aquaticus*) in 2018 (McAllister et al., 2018). However, the molecular characteristic data of *Cyclospora* in other animals, including *Cyclospora* in vipers, moles, myriapodes, rodents were largely absent. More research work is needed to supplement the missing data in the future.

2.3 Genome characteristics

2.3.1 Mitochondrial genome

The mitochondrial genome of *C. cayetanensis* is approximately 6200 bp in length, with 33% GC content (Cinar et al., 2015; Ogedengbe et al., 2015; Tang et al., 2015). It codes 3 protein-coding genes (*cytb*, *cox1*, and *cox3*), 14 large subunit (LSU), and 9 small subunit (SSU) fragmented rRNA genes (Cinar et al., 2015; Ogedengbe et al., 2015). The mitochondrial genome of *C. cayetanensis* has a linear concatemer or circular mapping topology (Tang et al., 2015). Comparative genomic analysis showed high similarity between the *C. cayetanensis* and *Eimeria tenella* genomes, with 90.4% nucleotide sequence similarity and complete synteny in gene organization (Tang et al., 2015). Phylogenetic analysis of the mitochondrial genomic sequences has confirmed the genetic similarities between avian *Eimeria* spp. and *C. cayetanensis*.

In the phylum Apicomplexa, mitochondrial genomes have either concatemeric or monomeric linear structures, it was consistent with a concatemeric structure that is the hallmark of the closely related *Eimeria* mt genomes; however, it cannot rule out a circular mt genome structure. The complete *C. cayetanensis* mt genome is 6274 bp, with a base composition of A (30%), T (36%), C (16%), and G (17%). Based on the available annotations in the NCBI for *Eimeria gallopavonis*, *Cyclospora* mitochondrian genome was annotated after aligning the two genomes (Cinar et al., 2015). The *C. cayetanensis* mt genome encodes three protein-coding genes; cytb, 1080 bp [128–1207 bp], ATG start codon; cox1, 1443 bp [1248–2690 bp], GTT start codon; and cox3, 780 bp [4226–5005 bp], ATT start codon. In addition to these three protein-coding genes, 12 large-subunit (LSU) and 7 small-subunit (SSU) fragmented rRNA genes are present in the mt genome. Pairwise amino acid sequence alignments between the individual protein coding genes of *C. cayetanensis* mt genome and the corresponding coding genes of 17 other published *Eimeria* mt genomes revealed sequence identities that ranged from 90% to 97% for cytbB gene, 93% to 97% for cox1 gene, and 83% to 93% for cox3 gene.

Mitochondrial genomes of some *Eimeria* species were aligned with the *C. cayetanensis* mt genome for neighbor-joining (NJ) phylogenetic reconstruction analysis (Fig. 2.2). The mt genome nucleotide phylogeny of *C. cayetanensis* exhibited a closer relationship to *Eimeria* species (*E. magna* and *E. dispersa* that infect rabbits and turkeys, respectively). *C. cayetanensis* appears to infect only humans, and, notably, *C. cayetanensis* mt sequences fall into a clade that contains rabbit-infecting *E. magna* (Fig. 2.2). Avian-infecting *Eimeria* species in our comparison is clustered into two other distinct clades (Fig. 2.2). The monophyletic grouping of mammalian Coccidians (*Cyclospora* and *E. magna*) into mitochondrial phylogenetic tree warrants further analysis, preferably using apicomplexan apicoplastic and chromosomal genome sequences.

Blast analysis indicated that *C. cayetanensis* has 87%–92% sequence similarities to the mitochondrial genomes of various *Eimeria* spp. in GenBank, with the highest similarity to the genome in *E. dispersa* (KJ608416). This was confirmed by direct comparison of the assembled *C. cayetanensis* and *E. tenella* genomes by using NUCmer, which showed an overall sequence identity of 90.4%. Comparison of the mitochondrial genomes of apicomplexans indicated that the *C. cayetanensis* genome has complete synteny with genomes of *Eimeria* spp. Analysis of SNV distribution by read mapping along the genome of *E. tenella* showed that the most conserved regions are nucleotide positions 2800–4900 and positions 5400 to the end of the genome, where the rRNA gene fragments are located. Phylogenetic analysis of the mitochondrial genome sequences demonstrated that *C. cayetanensis*

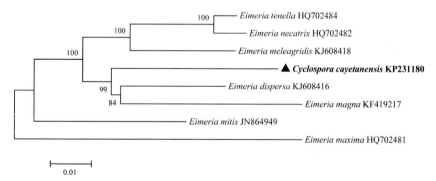

Fig. 2.2 Phylogenetic relationship between *C. cayetanensis* and other apicomplexan protozoa. Phylogeny inferred with a neighbor-joining analysis of mitochondrial genomes (B) reported by Cinar et al. (2015), based on distances calculated with the Kimura 2-parameter model. Bootstrap values >50% from 1000 replicates are shown at the nodes. Scale bars indicate estimated substitutions per site.

formed a clade with *E. dispersa* from turkeys and quails and *E. magna* from rabbits, sister to a clade formed by cecum-infecting *Eimeria* spp. from chickens and turkeys.

2.3.2 Apicoplast genome

The apicoplast genome of *C. cayetanensis* is approximately 34,000 bp in size and codes 65 genes, with 22% GC content (Tang et al., 2015; Liu et al., 2016). The apicoplast genome is circular, codes the complete machinery for protein biosynthesis, and contains two inverted repeats that differ slightly in LSU rRNA gene sequences (Tang et al., 2015). Comparative genomic analysis revealed high nucleotide sequence similarity (85.6%) between *C. cayetanensis* and *E. tenella*. Phylogenetic analysis of the apicoplast genomic sequences has also confirmed the genetic similarities between avian *Eimeria* spp. and *C. cayetanensis* (Fig. 2.3).

The apicoplast genome is 34,155 bp in size with the following base composition: A—40.28%, T—37.76%, C—10.79%), and G—11.16%), with an overall GC content of 21.96%. It contained two inverted repeats (IR). Each IR unit is 5244 bp in length and contains genes coding for an SSU rRNA, an LSU rRNA, and nine tRNAs. The annotation of the sequences indicated that there are 65 genes coded by the apicoplast genome, including 4 rRNA genes, 28 protein-coding genes, and 33 tRNA genes for all 20 amino acids. The protein-coding genes include 6 genes for ribosomal protein large subunit (rpl), 10 genes for ribosomal protein small subunit (rps), 3 genes for RNA polymerase (rpo), 6 genes for hypothetical proteins, and 1 gene each for elongation factor Tu (tufA), ATP-dependent Clp protease (clpC), and putative ABC transporter (ycf24). The *C. cayetanensis* apicoplast has almost all the genes

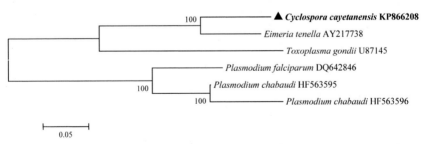

Fig. 2.3 Phylogenetic relationship between *C. cayetanensis* and other apicomplexan protozoa. Phylogeny inferred with a neighbor-joining analysis of apicoplast genomes (C) reported by Tang et al. (2015), based on distances calculated with the Kimura 2-parameter model. Bootstrap values >50% from 1000 replicates are shown at the nodes. Scale bars indicate estimated substitutions per site.

encoded in the *E. tenella* apicoplast genome except rpl36, which is truncated. Similarly, the orf-D gene of *C. cayetanensis* codes for only 70 amino acids in length, which is 29 amino acids shorter than that of *E. tenella*. Orf-A codes for a protein similar to the DNA-directed RNA polymerase subunit.

A BLAST search of the NCBI database with the *C. cayetanensis* apicoplast sequence showed that the sequence was most similar to the apicoplast genome of *E. tenella* (access no. AY217738). Genome sequence alignments show that the *C. cayetanensis* apicoplast genome has complete gene synteny to the apicoplast genome of *E. tenella* and other *Eimeria* spp. and good synteny to the genome of *T. gondii*. Aligning the assembled apicoplast genome sequence to that of the *E. tenella* apicoplast genome with NUCmer resulted in a single alignment that covers 99.85% of the apicoplast genome, confirming the synteny between the two genomes. The identity between the two genomes in the aligned regions was 85.6%. The sequence divergence between the two genomes was mostly 8%–10% as calculated in a sliding window of 1000 bp in sequence read mapping. However, much lower sequence differences were seen in rRNA genes within the two IR units. SNV analysis by read mapping did not identify any intraisolate sequence polymorphism beyond what was described between the two IRs.

In a neighbor-joining analysis of apicoplast genome sequences from apicomplexans, *C. cayetanensis*, *E. tenella* formed one clade that was divergent from *T. gondii* and *Plasmodium* spp. Within the clade formed by *Cyclospora* and *Eimeria*, *C. cayetanensis* clustered together with *E. tenella*, confirming the genetic similarity between the two species based on direct sequence comparison and gene annotations.

2.3.3 Chromosome genome

The whole genome of *C. cayetanensis* has a total length of 44 Mbp, with 52% GC content, and codes 7457 genes (Liu et al., 2016). Comparative genomic analysis indicates that *C. cayetanensis* shares coccidia-like metabolism and invasion components but has unique surface antigens (Liu et al., 2016). In addition, there are some major differences in the amino acid metabolism and posttranslation modification of proteins between *C. cayetanensis* and other apicomplexans (Liu et al., 2016). A multilocus sequence typing (MLST) tool for *C. cayetanensis* have been developed based on its whole genome, involving five microsatellite loci (Guo et al., 2016). Noticeable geographic clustering is observed in human *C. cayetanensis* isolates from around the world (Li et al., 2017). This could be useful for case linkage and tracking of cyclosporiasis outbreaks.

It obtained a draft genome of *C. cayetanensis* with a total length of 44,034,550 bp. The genome of *C. cayetanensis* is slightly smaller than genomes of *T. gondii* and *E. tenella*. Altogether, 74.4% of the core eukaryotic protein-encoding genes were covered by the genome of *C. cayetanensis*, which is comparable to that of whole genome sequences from *T. gondii* (85.1%) and *E. tenella* (68.1%). It has a gene density similar to that of *E. tenella* and *T. gondii*, but lower than that seen in some other apicomplexan parasites.

The alternation of repeat-rich and repeat-poor regions, which was reported for *Eimeria* spp., was also detected in the *C. cayetanensis* genome. There are 87 putative long terminal repeat (LTR) retrotransposons in the *C. cayetanensis* genome. The length of putative LTRs in *C. cayetanensis* varies from 106 to 996 bp with an average of 337 bp, and the sequence similarity between upstream and downstream LTRs of each retrotransposon varies from 85.0% to 98.6%. Cluster analysis show that they could be divided into 44 types based on sequence identities. Unlike *Eimeria* spp., whose LTR retrotransposons belong to chromoviruses, neither the chromodomain nor the functional domain of reverse transcriptases was identified in LTR retrotransposons of *C. cayetanensis*.

There are 144 predicted tRNA genes in the *C. cayetanensis* genome, which is slightly less than that in *T. gondii* (174) but much higher than that in other apicomplexans. It identified 11 rRNA genes in the draft genome of *C. cayetanensis*. The *C. cayetanensis* genome may encode as many as 7457 proteins. Among them, 538 proteins have signal peptides (105 of them target the apicoplast), 1247 had one or more transmembrane regions, and 225 had a GPIanchor attachment site. These numbers are similar to those in *E. tenella* and *T. gondii*. All orthologs of bacterial genes found in *C. cayetanensis* are also present in other apicomplexans, implying a possible origin through lateral gene transfer. Pfam searching indicates that a large group (~1020) of functional domains is shared by apicomplexans and a smaller group (~546) by coccidia. The heteroxenous *T. gondii* apparently possesses more unique protein domains than the monoxenous *E. tenella* and *C. cayetanensis*.

Tracing the source of infection can be facilitated by genomic comparison between isolates. Moreover, *Cyclospora* may be clearly identified and differentiated from other protozoan parasites involved in foodborne or waterborne outbreaks by genomic difference.

2.4 Case-linking and tracking

Numerous *C. cayetanensis* genotyping methods have been developed, and they are useful for epidemiological trace-back investigations of cyclosporiasis (Cinar et al., 2020). For case-linking and transmission source tracking, a multilocus sequence typing (MLST) tool has been established for *C. cayetanensis* that involves five microsatellite loci (Guo et al., 2016). There are also other potential uses for this MLST tool (Hofstetter et al., 2019). It has been used to investigate *C. cayetanensis* genetic population characterization (Li et al., 2017; Guo et al., 2018). Recently, qPCR (Guo et al., 2019) and standard PCR assays (Nascimento et al., 2019) have been developed for the genotyping of *C. cayetanensis* that use the polymorphic region by using targeted enrichment of complete mitochondrial genomes and next-generation sequencing (Cinar et al., 2020). Relationships have been corroborated by a significant number of epidemiological linkages, suggesting the usefulness of the technique for aiding epidemiological trace-back, case-linkage, source-tracking, and distinct case cluster investigations (Barratt et al., 2019; Guo et al., 2019; Nascimento et al., 2019), especially during cyclosporiasis outbreaks.

2.5 Conclusion

Molecular genotyping, using targeted amplicon sequencing, provides a complementary tool for cyclosporiasis outbreak investigations, especially when epidemiological data are insufficient for linking cases and identifying clusters. Characteristics of polymorphic regions of the *Cyclospora* genome had been studied to better understand the microorganism's mode of infection and molecular epidemiology. The molecular typing of *C. cayetanensis* in produce and clinical samples by using targeted enrichment of complete genomes and next-generation sequencing can distinguish between distinct case clusters and might be helpful during cyclosporiasis outbreak investigations.

References

Adam, R.D., Ortega, Y.R., Gilman, R.H., Sterling, C.R., 2000. Intervening transcribed spacer region 1 variability in *Cyclospora cayetanensis*. J. Clin. Microbiol. 38, 2339–2343.

Almeria, S., Cinar, H.N., Dubey, J.P., 2019. *Cyclospora cayetanensis* and cyclosporiasis: an update. Microorganisms 7, 317.

Barratt, J.L.N., Park, S., Nascimento, F.S., Hofstetter, J., Plucinski, M., Casillas, S., Bradbury, R.S., Arrowood, M.J., Qvarnstrom, Y., Talundzic, E., 2019. Genotyping genetically heterogeneous *Cyclospora cayetanensis* infections to complement epidemiological case linkage. Parasitology 146, 1275–1283.

Buss, S.N., Leber, A., Chapin, K., Fey, P.D., Bankowski, M.J., Jones, M.K., Rogatcheva, M., Kanack, K.J., Bourzac, K.M., 2015. Multicenter evaluation of the BioFire FilmArray gastrointestinal panel for etiologic diagnosis of infectious gastroenteritis. J. Clin. Microbiol. 53, 915–925.

Cinar, H.N., Gopinath, G., Jarvis, K., Murphy, H.R., 2015. The complete mitochondrial genome of the foodborne parasitic pathogen *Cyclospora cayetanensis*. PLoS One 10, e0128645.

Cinar, H.N., Gopinath, G., Murphy, H.R., Almeria, S., Durigan, M., Choi, D., Jang, A., Kim, E., Kim, R., Choi, S., Lee, J., Shin, Y., Lee, J., Qvarnstrom, Y., Benedict, T.K., Bishop, H.S., da Silva, A., 2020. Molecular typing of *Cyclospora cayetanensis* in produce and clinical samples using targeted enrichment of complete mitochondrial genomes and next-generation sequencing. Parasit. Vectors 13, 122.

Eberhard, M.L., da Silva, A.J., Lilley, B.G., Pieniazek, N.J., 1999. Morphologic and molecular characterization of new *Cyclospora* species from Ethiopian monkeys: *C. cercopitheci* sp.n., *C. colobi* sp.n., and *C. papionis* sp.n. Emerg. Infect. Dis., 651–658.

Guo, Y., Roellig, D.M., Li, N., Tang, K., Frace, M., Ortega, Y., Arrowood, M.J., Feng, Y., Qvarnstrom, Y., Wang, L., Moss, D.M., Zhang, L., Xiao, L., 2016. Multilocus sequence typing tool for *Cyclospora cayetanensis*. Emerg. Infect. Dis. 22, 1464–1467.

Guo, Y., Li, N., Ortega, Y.R., Zhang, L., Roellig, D.M., Feng, Y., Xiao, L., 2018. Population genetic characterization of *Cyclospora cayetanensis* from discrete geographical regions. Exp. Parasitol. 184, 121–127.

Guo, Y., Wang, Y., Wang, X., Zhang, L., Ortega, Y., Feng, Y., 2019. Mitochondrial genome sequence variation as a useful marker for assessing genetic heterogeneity among *Cyclospora cayetanensis* isolates and source-tracking. Parasit. Vectors 12, 47.

Hannet, I., Engsbro, A.L., Pareja, J., Schneider, U.V., Lisby, J.G., Pružinec-Popović, B., Hoerauf, A., Parčina, M., 2019. Multicenter evaluation of the new QIAstat gastrointestinal panel for the rapid syndromic testing of acute gastroenteritis. Eur. J. Clin. Microbiol. Infect. Dis. 38, 2103–2112.

Hitchcock, M.M., Hogan, C.A., Budvytiene, I., Banaei, N., 2019. Reproducibility of positive results for rare pathogens on the FilmArray GI panel. Diagn. Microbiol. Infect. Dis. 95, 10–14.

Hofstetter, J.N., Nascimento, F.S., Park, S., Casillas, S., Herwaldt, B.L., Arrowood, M.J., Qvarnstrom, Y., 2019. Evaluation of multilocus sequence typing of *Cyclospora cayetanensis* based on microsatellite markers. Parasite 26, 3.

Li, J., Sun, F., Wang, R., Zhang, L., 2015a. Advances in research on food-borne infection and detection methods of *Cyclospora*. Food Sci. 36, 261–267.

Li, N., Ye, J., Arrowood, M.J., Ma, J., Wang, L., Xu, H., Feng, Y., Xiao, L., 2015b. Identification and morphologic and molecular characterization of *Cyclospora macacae* n. sp. from rhesus monkeys in China. Parasitol. Res. 114, 1811–1816.

Li, J., Chang, Y., Shi, K.E., Wang, R., Fu, K., Li, S., Xu, J., Jia, L., Guo, Z., Zhang, L., 2017. Multilocus sequence typing and clonal population genetic structure of *Cyclospora cayetanensis* in humans. Parasitology 144, 1890–1897.

Li, J., Wang, R., Chen, Y., Xiao, L., Zhang, L., 2020. *Cyclospora cayetanensis* infection in humans: biological characteristics, clinical features, epidemiology, detection method, and treatment. Parasitology 147, 160–170.

Liu, S., Wang, L., Zheng, H., Xu, Z., Roellig, D.M., Li, N., Frace, M.A., Tang, K., Arrowood, M.J., Moss, D.M., Zhang, L., Feng, Y., Xiao, L., 2016. Comparative genomics reveals

Cyclospora cayetanensis possesses coccidia-like metabolism and invasion components but unique surface antigens. BMC Genomics 17, 316.

McAllister, C.T., Motriuk-Smith, D., Kerr, C.M., 2018. Three new coccidians (*Cyclospora, Eimeria*) from eastern moles, *Scalopus aquaticus* (Linnaeus) (Mammalia: Soricomorpha: Talpidae) from Arkansas, USA. Syst. Parasitol. 95, 271–279.

Nascimento, F.S., Barta, J.R., Whale, J., Hofstetter, J.N., Casillas, S., Barratt, J., Talundzic, E., Arrowood, M.J., Qvarnstrom, Y., 2019. Mitochondrial junction region as genotyping marker for *Cyclospora cayetanensis*. Emerg. Infect. Dis. 25, 1314–1319.

Ogedengbe, M.E., Qvarnstrom, Y., da Silva, A.J., Arrowood, M.J., Barta, J.R., 2015. A linear mitochondrial genome of *Cyclospora cayetanensis* (Eimeriidae, Eucoccidiorida, Coccidiasina, Apicomplexa) suggests the ancestral start position within mitochondrial genomes of eimeriid coccidia. Int. J. Parasitol. 45, 361–365.

Olivier, C., van de Pas, S., Lepp, P.W., Yoder, K., Relman, D.A., 2001. Sequence variability in the first internal transcribed spacer region within and among *Cyclospora* species is consistent with polyparasitism. Int. J. Parasitol. 31, 1475–1487.

Relman, D.A., Schmidt, T.M., Gajadhar, A., Sogin, M., Cross, J., Yoder, K., Sethabutr, O., Echeverria, P., 1996. Molecular phylogenetic analysis of *Cyclospora*, the human intestinal pathogen, suggests that it is closely related to *Eimeria* species. J. Infect. Dis. 173, 440–445.

Riner, D.K., Nichols, T., Lucas, S.Y., Mullin, A.S., Cross, J.H., Lindquist, H.D., 2010. Intragenomic sequence variation of the ITS-1 region within a single flow-cytometry-counted *Cyclospora cayetanensis* oocysts. J. Parasitol. 96, 914–919.

Ryan, U., Paparini, A., Oskam, C., 2017. New technologies for detection of enteric parasites. Trends Parasitol. 33, 532–546.

Shin, J.H., Lee, S.E., Kim, T.S., Ma, D.W., Cho, S.H., Chai, J.Y., Shin, E.H., 2018. Development of molecular diagnosis using multiplex real-time PCR and T4 phage internal control to simultaneously detect *Cryptosporidium parvum, Giardia lamblia*, and *Cyclospora* cayetanensis from human stool samples. Korean J. Parasitol. 56, 419–427.

Sulaiman, I.M., Torres, P., Simpson, S., Kerdahi, K., Ortega, Y., 2013. Sequence characterization of heat shock protein gene of *Cyclospora cayetanensis* isolates from Nepal, Mexico, and Peru. J. Parasitol. 99, 379–382.

Sulaiman, I.M., Ortega, Y., Simpson, S., Kerdahi, K., 2014. Genetic characterization of human-pathogenic *Cyclospora cayetanensis* parasites from three endemic regions at the 18S ribosomal RNA locus. Infect. Genet. Evol. 22, 229–234.

Tang, K., Guo, Y., Zhang, L., Rowe, L.A., Roellig, D.M., Frace, M.A., Li, N., Liu, S., Feng, Y., Xiao, L., 2015. Genetic similarities between *Cyclospora cayetanensis* and cecum-infecting avian *Eimeria* spp. in apicoplast and mitochondrial genomes. Parasit. Vectors 8, 358.

Taniuchi, M., Verweij, J.J., Sethabutr, O., Bodhidatta, L., Garcia, L., Maro, A., Kumburu, H., Gratz, J., Kibiki, G., Houpt, E.R., 2011. Multiplex polymerase chain reaction method to detect *Cyclospora, Cystoisospora*, and microsporidia in stool samples. Diagn. Microbiol. Infect. Dis. 71, 386–390.

Varma, M., Hester, J.D., Schaefer 3rd, F.W., Ware, M.W., Lindquist, H.D., 2003. Detection of *Cyclospora cayetanensis* using a quantitative real-time PCR assay. J. Microbiol. Methods 53, 27–36.

CHAPTER 3

Clinical feature

Contents

3.1 Introduction

Cyclosporiasis, a protracted, relapsing gastroenteritis caused by *Cyclospora* spp., is associated with diarrhea among children in developing countries where *Cyclospora cayetanensis* is endemic, traveler's diarrhea, and/or sometimes foodborne and waterborne outbreaks in the developed countries (Chacín-Bonilla, 2010; Helmy, 2010). Of the 22 *Cyclospora* species identified in humans and animals till today (Ortega and Sanchez, 2010), *C. cayetanensis* is the only known species infecting humans reported in 56 countries worldwide, with the total prevalence of 3.55% (Li et al., 2020b). Human infection of *C. cayetanensis* is most commonly found in subtropical and tropical regions (Herwaldt, 2000), while cases in industrialized countries (e.g., North America and the United Kingdom) are frequently associated with the intake of contaminated food (especially small fruits, mixed salad greens, and herbs) (Milord et al., 2012) or travelers returning from tropical and/or developing countries (Li et al., 2020a). Although asymptomatic persons are more frequent in disease-endemic areas, cyclosporiasis, caused by *C. cayetanensis*, can be severe in both immunocompetent and immunocompromised individuals (Herwaldt, 2000; Zar et al., 2001). Clinically, profuse watery diarrhea is the typical manifestation of cyclosporiasis patients, and would also be accompanied by other alimentary and general symptoms (Shields and Olson, 2003; Li et al., 2020a, b), causing significant influence on the quality of patients' life. Further, *C. cayetanensis* or *Cyclospora*-like organism has been detected in the fecal samples of several animal species, e.g., chickens, dogs, ducks, cattle, sheep, goats, rats, house mice, birds, shellfish, drills (*Mandrillus leucophaeus poensis*), and nonhuman primates (Katz and Taylor, 2001; Zhao et al., 2013; Li et al., 2007, 2017, 2020b; Basnett et al., 2018; Marangi et al., 2015; Ghimire and Bhattarai, 2019; Giangaspero and Gasser, 2019), and the oocysts of *C. cayetanensis* could be recovered from the Asian freshwater clam (*Corbicula fluminea*) by artificial contamination (Graczyk et al., 1998), challenging the general opinion that human is the only reservoir for *C. cayetanensis*. However, to date, there has been no direct clinical or histologic proof of *C. cayetanensis* in these animal hosts. Therefore, this chapter mainly focuses on the clinical and pathological features of cyclosporiasis in humans.

3.2 Clinical features

To comprehensively and globally review the clinical features of cyclosporiasis, a total of 718 literature published in PubMed within National Center for Biotechnology Information (NCBI) were obtained by search using the key word "*Cyclospora*," and cyclosporiasis cases with detailed description of clinical characters and English abstracts or full texts were included.

3.2.1 Intestinal infection

From these current literature, the clinical manifestations of *Cyclospora* infection in humans are closely associated with the host status (e.g., age, immunity), endemicity in a particular region, dietary habit and experience (especially eating raw fruits and vegetables such as raspberries, blackberries, and lettuce), travel history, season, and other yet known factors (Puente et al., 2006; Giangaspero and Gasser, 2019).

Although high frequency of asymptomatic infection was found in indigenous populations in some developing countries (e.g., Peru and Haiti), gastrointestinal (GI) symptoms were frequently described in cyclosporidiosis patients in tropical and subtropical areas, and travelers returning from these endemic regions in developed countries, especially in United States and European nations (Okhuysen, 2001; Giangaspero and Gasser, 2019). The prepatent period of cyclosporiasis is variable and rather short, lasting from 1 to 11 days (average = 7 days) (Okhuysen, 2001; Puente et al., 2006). Diarrhea is the most striking presentation of patients in sporadic cases and outbreaks of cyclosporidiosis, though, sometimes, it is not the initial symptom after the incubation period. *Cyclospora* was recognized as a human diarrheal agent when it was first documented in Papua New Guinea by Ashford (1979).

Subsequently, this pathogenic coccidian parasite has been reported in both immunocompetent and immunocompromised (e.g., HIV/AIDS, transplant recipients) patients, causing sporadic-to-frequent explosive diarrhea with or without mucus, pus, and blood (Chacín-Bonilla, 2010; Helmy, 2010). A 43-year-old immunocompetent man in France, returning from Southeast Asia, with a 15-day history of watery diarrhea was diagnosed with infection of *C. cayetanensis* (Pons et al., 2012). A previous epidemiological surveillance study showed that *Cyclospora* spp. was detected in 1.4% (3/221) of Polish immunocompetent patients with acute or chronic diarrhea returning from international journeys to hot climates (Kłudkowska et al., 2017). Fortunately, diarrhea caused by *C. cayetanensis* in these immunocompetent individuals is generally transient or mildly to moderately self-limited (Li et al., 2020a, b), characterized by nonbloody, watery diarrhea in a cyclical pattern, sometimes alternating with constipation (Mota et al., 2000), and lasting from 6 to 8 weeks (Looney, 1998).

Further, consequence of diarrhea is different by age (Almeria et al., 2019), and the duration and severity of disease decreases with aging for children in endemic areas (Ortega and Sanchez, 2010). That being said, elderly individual and younger children have more severe diarrhea (Ortega and Sanchez, 2010; Almeria et al., 2019), but diarrheic syndrome is rarely found in children within 3 years of age (Mota et al., 2000), while milder infection is seen in elder children and adults (Ortega and Sanchez, 2010; Almeria et al., 2019). Of 200 children (4–168 months) with diarrhea examined in All India Institute of Medical Sciences, New Delhi (India), irrespective of their immune status, 5 (2.5%) were positive for *Cyclospora* infection, with 2 as immunocompetent patients (Kumar et al., 2017). A study conducted in school children between 3 and 14 years of age in Kathmandu, Nepal in 2014 showed that 3.94% (20/507) of the stool samples were positive for *Cyclospora* infection, with high prevalence in students aged 3–5 years (10.15%) presenting with diarrheal symptoms (10.57%), followed by household keeping livestock (10.11%) and consumers of raw vegetables/fruits (7.25%) (Bhandari et al., 2015).

Notably, diarrhea associated with cyclosporiasis is more severe in immunocompromised or immunosuppressed patients and the duration of diarrhea is very long (Ortega and Sanchez, 2010; Almeria et al., 2019). A Poland businessman with renal transplant and having ongoing immunosuppressive treatment developed acute and prolonged diarrhea after returning from Indonesia (Bednarska et al., 2015). *C. cayetanensis* was also detected in transplant recipients presenting with diarrhea in India (Yadav et al., 2016).

A metadata analysis showed higher prevalence rates in immunocompromised persons, with the prevalence ranging from 0% to 36% (average 4.5%) among 3340 investigated immunocompromised persons (mostly HIV/AIDS patients with diarrhea) (Chacín-Bonilla, 2010). Significant differences in *Cyclospora* infection were found between HIV-seropositive and HIV-seronegative individuals in Nigeria (Udeh et al., 2019). Previous studies found longer average duration of diarrhea in HIV-positive patients compared with HIV-negative ones (Ortega and Sanchez, 2010), and the diarrhea in AIDS patients may persist for 12 weeks or more (Chawla and Ichhpujani, 2011). Patients with depletion of T cells and low number CD4$^+$ T cells have been reported at greater risk for infection of some opportunistic protozoa (e.g., *Cryptosporidium* spp.) (Marcos and Gotuzzo, 2013). Asma et al. (2011) investigated the intestinal parasitism in HIV-infected patients in Malaysia, and found that patients harboring intestinal parasites had significantly lower CD4 counts (i.e., 200 cells/mm^3). It is shocking that the CD4 counts in all the 14 *Cyclospora*-positive patients were 0–400 cells/mm^3 and half were lower than 400 cells/mm^3. In a study conducted in HIV-infected patients in Nepal, *Cyclospora* infection was only detected in participants with CD4 T-cell counts < 200/μL (Tiwari et al., 2013). The coinfection of *C. cayetanensis* and *Salmonella typhi* was found in an HIV patient with chronic diarrhea with a CD4 count of 130 cells/mm^3 (Llanes et al., 2013). However, some studies also found no significant correlations between *Cyclospora* infection and CD4 count (Nsagha et al., 2016; Zorbozan et al., 2018). Thus, more studies should be conducted to evident the effect of CD4 T-cell counts on *Cyclospora* infection.

In addition to diarrhea, other GI symptoms were also accompanied commonly or sometimes (Herwaldt and Ackers, 1997; Blans et al., 2005; Puente et al., 2006; Insulander et al., 2010; Milord et al., 2012; Orozco-Mosqueda et al., 2014), including stomach and abdominal pain or cramps, abdominal discomfort, vomiting, nausea or appetite loss or hyporexia, constipation or obstipation, abdominal bloating or gas or flatulence and abdominal distension, anorexia, increased peristalsis, anal pruritus, postprandial fullness, heart burn reflux, borborygmi, rectal tenesmus, and unintentional weight loss. Almost invariable loss in body weight was seen during untreated illness, with an average even up to 6–7 kg (Shlim, 2002). Malabsorption of D-xylose and increased excretion of fecal fat virtually always occur. Moreover, prodromal illness (flu-like) myalgias and arthralgias and constitutional symptoms (such as headache, fatigue, chills, usually low-grade fever, muscle, joint, or generalized body aches, malnutrition, general malaise, asthenia, eructation) could be seen in *Cyclospora*-positive patients, sometimes preceding the onset of GI symptoms (Karanja et al., 2007). For example, diarrhea and nausea were found in all 18 patients in a foodborne outbreak of *Cyclospora* infection in Stockholm, Sweden, followed by abdominal pain (75%), fever (66%), and vomiting (33%) (Insulander et al., 2010). In a point source outbreak acquired in Guatemala, diarrhea, asthenia, anorexia, borborygmi, flatulence, and abdominal distension were present in all the seven Spanish travelers (Puente et al., 2006). In a large outbreak in the United States in 1996, diarrhea together with anorexia, fatigue, and weight loss were the four most common symptoms, occurring in > 90% of case patients (Herwaldt and Ackers, 1997). Intriguingly, moderate weight losses (~3.5 kg) were observed in non-AIDS patients with *Cyclospora* infection, whereas more severe losses (~7.2 kg) were reported in AIDS patients (Ortega and Sanchez, 2010). Certainty, evidence of clinical symptoms but not diarrhea was also seen in some cases of *C. cayetanensis* infection. For example, a field survey conducted by the Faculty of Tropical Medicine, Mahidol University showed that of 12 schoolchildren cases aged 5–12 years, five had loose feces, one reported frequent symptoms of abdominal discomfort, and another had pale conjunctiva with low hematocrit (Thima et al., 2014).

Furthermore, intranuclear coccidiosis caused by *Cyclospora* spp. was reported in three castrated male Japanese Black calves from two farms in Oita Prefecture, Japan between 2010 and 2011 (Yamada et al., 2014). One case presented watery diarrhea, anorexia, and rough hair coat for 6 weeks, and the other two calves suffered from severe emaciation, with retardation and anorexia. Histologic examination and sequence analysis of parasite 18S ribosomal RNA showed the infection of *Cyclospora* spp. Although *Cyclospora* species were not identified, this study provided the clinical findings that suggest that it could be associated with *Cyclospora* infection in calves.

3.2.2 Extraintestinal infection

More strikingly, biliary disease is another clinical manifestation in AIDS patients infected with *C. cayetanensis*. To our best knowledge, *C. cayetanensis*-related clinical cholecystitis was reported in only four patients with AIDS (Sifuentes-Osornio et al., 1995; Zar et al., 2001; de Górgolas et al., 2001; Dubey et al., 2020). Between September 1993 and June 1994, of 235 patients with diarrheal disease (three or more loose or watery stools per day) at the Department of Infectious Diseases of the Instituto Nacional de la Nutricion Salvador Zubiran in Mexico, 2 cyclosporidiosis patients with AIDS had biliary disease, with distention and thickening of the gallbladder wall (a finding suggestive of acalculous cholecystitis) in both patients shown by ultrasonography (Sifuentes-Osornio et al., 1995). Zar et al. (2001) reported acalculous cholecystitis caused by *C. cayetanensis* in a 35-year-old HIV-positive man. In addition to a 10-day history of sudden onset of nonfoul-smelling watery diarrhea without blood or pus, he presented the onset of right upper quadrant pain that worsened with eating and radiated to the right subscapular region, and his temperature was up to 38.3°C (Zar et al., 2001). *C. cayetanensis* cholecystitis was also diagnosed in a 33-year-old man with AIDS from Honduras. Besides GI symptoms, acute right-upper-quadrant abdominal pain and fever were present.

Like other coccidian parasites (e.g., *Cryptosporidium* spp.), some sequelae such as Guillain-Barré syndrome (GBS) and reactive arthritis syndrome (formally Reiter syndrome) would be triggered due to prolonged infection of *C. cayetanensis* (Richardson et al., 1998; Connor et al., 2001; Sloan, 2001; Shields and Olson, 2003; Karanja et al., 2007). A 58-year-old, right-handed hypertensive man with diarrhea and fever (38.6°C) was diagnosed with infection of *C. cayetanensis*. He was then quadriparetic, areflexic, and mechanically ventilated within 18 h of admission. Serial nerve conduction studies indicated common pattern of GBS, and circumstantial evidence suggests *C. cayetanensis* was another trigger for GBS presumably by inducing immune response (Richardson et al., 1998). A 31-year-old man infected with *Cyclospora* was allergic to sulfa and thus could not be treated with standard therapy-trimethoprim/sulfamethoxazole (TMP-SMX); the patient then developed Reiter syndrome presenting ocular inflammation, inflammatory oligoarthritis, and sterile urethritis (Connor et al., 2001).

Curiously, the acid-fast *C. cayetanensis* oocysts were observed in sputum samples of two HIV-negative patients (Di Gliullo et al., 2000; Hussein et al., 2005). One patient was a 60-year-old man and was successfully treated for pulmonary tuberculosis during 1997, but he presented symptoms such as loss of weight, cough with purulent expectoration, dysphonia, and a radiological picture of pulmonary fibrosis (Di Gliullo et al., 2000). Large (8–10 μm) spherical, acid-fast *C. cayetanensis* oocysts were found in sputum stained with Ziehl-Neelsen technique. Another case was that of a 45-years-old male patient with active pulmonary tuberculosis in Ismailia of Egypt, presenting loss of weight, cough with expectoration of purulent sputum, and dyspnea (Hussein et al., 2005). The infection of *C. cayetanensis* was confirmed in sputum samples by using Ziehl-Neelsen stain technique and nested PCR. Fortunately, there has been no direct evidence to show parasitism and harm of *C. cayetanensis* in the human respiratory system. However, these findings suggest that *C. cayetanensis* should be considered in the differential diagnosis with infections of other respiratory pathogens, and further studies on correlation between pulmonary tuberculosis and cyclosporidiosis should also be conducted in the future.

3.3 Pathological features

After ingestion by hosts, sporocysts released from *Cyclospora* oocysts inhabit the upper small intestine (preferably the jejunum), initiate the infection, and spent the intermediary stages of life cycle in the cytoplasma of enterocytes (Bintsis, 2017), responsible for acute and chronic inflammatory lesions in the epithelium, mucosa, and lamina propria; villous atrophy; and crypt hyperplasia (Mota et al., 2000).

In 1993, Connor and his colleagues reported pathological changes in the small bowel in nine diarrheal patients associated with a coccidian-like body (now called *Cyclospora*) (Connor et al., 1993). Of them, five had endoscopic evidence of moderate to marked erythema of distal duodenum. Histopathological findings suggested surface epithelial injury, especially near the tips of the villi, with focal vacuolization, loss of brush border, and an alteration of cells from a columnar to a cuboidal shape. Varying degrees of villous atrophy and crypt hyperplasia were found, with shortened, blunted villi and increased crypt length and mitoses. Further observation on endoscopic duodenal biopsies showed mild to moderate acute inflammation of the lamina propria and diffuse chronic inflammation in all cases. The plasma cells increased in the lamina propria and intraepithelial lymphocytes were focally elevated. Five of them also had neutrophils in the epithelium. Surprisingly, *Cyclospora* oocysts but not parasitic vacuoles were detected in duodenal aspirates of two patients. In the same year, CLB was found in jejunal aspirates in two of three male patients, and electronmicroscopic observation showed that it was located inside a vacuole within the cytoplasm of epithelial cells, and asexual stages (e.g., binucleate parasites) of this parasite were also seen in jejunal biopsy specimens (Bendall et al., 1993). Conventional HE staining of jejunal biopsy specimens showed jejunitis with increased intraepithelial leucocytes and villous blunting and fusion (Bendall et al., 1993).

Subsequently, *Cyclospora* oocysts and four asexual forms (sporozoite, trophozoite, schizont, and merozoite) within parasitophorous vacuoles located in the apical supranuclear region of enterocytes were clearly documented in a duodenal biopsy specimen of a 43-year-old HIV-positive Hispanic man with watery diarrhea (Sun et al., 1996). The lamina propria in the duodenum was expanded due to an infiltrate of lymphocytes and plasma cells, and oocysts were evident only within enterocytes of mucosal villi in the duodenum, but not in the stomach, transverse and sigmoid colon, and rectum (Sun et al., 1996). Supranuclear intracytoplasmic vacuoles with 6–8 comma-shaped structures (merozoites) were also found in duodenal enterocytes lining the mucosal villi in a 38-year-old HIV-seropositive man with *Cyclospora* infection, and an above-normal number of plasmocytic cells in the lamina propria (Deluol et al., 1996). Regrettably, the sexual stages were not identified in these studies. However, interestingly, *Cyclospora* oocytes were detected in stools of patients with asexual stages (Deluol et al., 1996; Sun et al., 1996), suggesting sexual cycle took place in humans and *Cyclospora* could complete its entire life cycle in only one host. In 1997, both asexual (two different types of meronts containing fully mature merozoites) and sexual (macrogametocytes) forms of *Cyclospora* organisms within parasitophorous vacuoles were found at the luminal surface and in the glandular clefts of human jejunum (Ortega et al., 1997).

Further, an altered mucosal architecture was observed in jejunal biopsies, with dramatic shortening and widening of the intestinal villi. Diffuse edema and mixed inflammatory cell infiltration were also detected, including plasma cells, lymphocytes, and eosinophils. Additionally, reactive hyperemia with vascular dilatation and congestion of villous capillaries were present, and moderate to marked erythema of the distal duodenum and mild to moderate acute inflammation of the lamina propria were found. However, no gross abnormalities (such as ulcers or hemorrhages) were identified in the stomachs and small intestines of patients. In 1999, merogony/schizogony of *Cyclospora* organisms and varying degrees of gross and microscopic gastrointestinal inflammation were evident in three healthy immunocompetent patients with symptomatic *C. cayetanensis* infection (Connor et al., 1999). Most strikingly, an electron-dense phospholipid membrane/myelin-like material (MLM) accumulated between the base and sides of enterocytes in two patients, with the presence of MLM both before and after treatment in one patient, and the amount of MLM was seemed to be associated with prolonged disease (Connor et al., 1999), suggesting MLM as a possible marker for cell injury, especially for persistent inflammation.

In addition to pathological lesions in human small intestine, histopathological proof was also obtained in the gallbladder of cyclosporosis patients with infection of HIV (Sifuentes-Osornio et al., 1995; Zar et al., 2001; de Górgolas et al., 2001; Dubey et al., 2020). Ultrasonography showed thickening of the gallbladder wall in two cyclosporosis patients with biliary disease, and the gallbladder wall in both patients returned to its normal thickness after the initiation of treatment with TMP-SMZ (Sifuentes-Osornio et al., 1995). However, no direct evidence for biliary infection due to *Cyclospora* was found in these patients. In 2001, an ultrasound on the right upper quadrant of a 35-year-old man infected with *C. cayetanensis* showed thickening of the anterior portion of the gallbladder wall but with no stones, pericholecystic fluid, or dilation of the bile ducts, while acute and chronic cholecystitis were identified in routine histologic sections of gallbladder (Zar et al., 2001). Numerous *Cyclospora* asexual forms (trophozoite, merozoite, and schizont) were found within intracytoplasmic parasitophorous vacuoles in the gallbladder epithelium, and *Cyclospora* oocysts were also demonstrated in the gallbladder epithelium by using auramine-rhodamine fluorochrome staining. In 2020, details of endogenous developmental cycle of *C. cayetanensis* were reported in the gallbladder of a 33-year-old man infected with HIV (Dubey et al., 2020). All stages were seen in the host epithelial cell cytoplasm within a parasitophorous vacuole, including immature and mature asexual schizonts, gamonts, and oocysts. Ultrasonography showed an enlarged gallbladder with a thickened wall, without gallstones, and thickening of the common biliary duct. An edematous intrahepatic bile tree in the abdomen was also indicted by using computed tomography (de Górgolas et al., 2001; Dubey et al., 2020).

3.4 Conclusion

Since first report of *C. cayetanensis* infection in Papua New Guinea in 1979, great progress has been achieved in revealing the clinical and pathological features of *Cyclospora* infection in immunocompetent and immunocompromise humans worldwide. *Cyclospora* infection could cause gastrointestinal and extragastrointestinal (mainly gallbladder) sequela, and would also be accompanied by general symptoms. However, our understanding on pathogenesis of *Cyclospora* still has a very long way to go. For example, mechanisms of *Cyclospora* causing diarrhea are not fully explored; the way by which sporozoites travel from the intestinal lumen to bile ducts initiating the development of *Cyclospora* is still unclear; the parasitism and damage of *Cyclospora* in human respiratory system are unresolved; the parasitism and pathogenicity of *C. cayetanensis* to hosts other than humans should be studied; the role of *Cyclospora* dense MLM during infection and clearance is unknown. Issues including but not limited to the points addressed will open a new perspective for the control of *Cyclospora* infection in humans as well as other hosts.

References

Almeria, S., Cinar, H.N., Dubey, J.P., 2019. *Cyclospora cayetanensis* and Cyclosporiasis: an update. Microorganisms 7 (9), 317.

Ashford, R.W., 1979. Occurrence of an undescribed coccidian in man in Papua New Guinea. Ann. Trop. Med. Parasitol. 73, 497–500.

Asma, I., Johari, S., Sim, B.L., Lim, Y.A., 2011. How common is intestinal parasitism in HIV-infected patients in Malaysia? Trop. Biomed. 28 (2), 400–410.

Basnett, K., Nagarajan, K., Soundararajan, C., Vairamuthu, S., Rao, G.V.S., 2018. Morphological and molecular identification of *Cyclospora* species in sheep and goat at Tamil Nadu, India. J. Parasit. Dis. 42 (4), 604–607.

Bednarska, M., Bajer, A., Welc-Falęciak, R., Pawełas, A., 2015. *Cyclospora cayetanensis* infection in transplant traveller: a case report of outbreak. Parasit. Vectors 8, 411.

Bendall, R.P., Lucas, S., Moody, A., Tovey, G., Chiodini, P.L., 1993. Diarrhoea associated with cyanobacterium-like bodies: a new coccidian enteritis of man. Lancet 341 (8845), 590–592.

Bhandari, D., Tandukar, S., Parajuli, H., Thapa, P., Chaudhary, P., Shrestha, D., Shah, P.K., Sherchan, J.B., Sherchand, J.B., 2015. *Cyclospora* infection among school children in Kathmandu, Nepal: prevalence and associated risk factors. Trop. Med. Health 43 (4), 211–216.

Bintsis, T., 2017. Foodborne pathogens. AIMS Microbiol. 3 (3), 529–563.

Blans, M.C., Ridwan, B.U., Verweij, J.J., Rozenberg-Arska, M., Verhoef, J., 2005. Cyclosporiasis outbreak, Indonesia. Emerg. Infect. Dis. 11 (9), 1453–1455.

Chacín-Bonilla, L., 2010. Epidemiology of *Cyclospora* cayetanensis: a review focusing in endemic areas. Acta Trop. 115 (3), 181–193.

Chawla, R., Ichhpujani, R.L., 2011. Enteric spore-forming opportunistic parasites in HIV/AIDS. Trop. Parasitol. 1 (1), 15–19.

Connor, B.A., Shlim, D.R., Scholes, J.V., Rayburn, J.L., Reidy, J., Rajah, R., 1993. Pathologic changes in the small bowel in nine patients with diarrhea associated with a coccidia-like body. Ann. Intern. Med. 119 (5), 377–382.

Connor, B.A., Reidy, J., Soave, R., 1999. Cyclosporiasis: clinical and histopathologic correlates. Clin. Infect. Dis. 28 (6), 1216–1222.

Connor, B.A., Johnson, E.J., Soave, R., 2001. Reiter syndrome following protracted symptoms of *Cyclospora* infection. Emerg. Infect. Dis. 7 (3), 453–454.

de Górgolas, M., Fortés, J., Fernández Guerrero, M.L., 2001. *Cyclospora cayetanensis* Cholecystitis in a patient with AIDS. Ann. Intern. Med. 134 (2), 166.

Deluol, A.M., Teilhac, M.F., Poirot, J.L., Heyer, F., Beaugerie, L., Chatelet, F.P., 1996. *Cyclospora* sp: life cycle studies in patient by electron-microscopy. J. Eukaryot. Microbiol. 43 (5), 128S–129S.

Di Gliullo, A.B., Cribari, M.S., Bava, A.J., Cicconetti, J.S., Collazos, R., 2000. *Cyclospora cayetanensis* in sputum and stool samples. Rev. Inst. Med. Trop. Sao Paulo 42 (2), 115–117.

Dubey, J.P., Almeria, S., Mowery, J., Fortes, J., 2020. Endogenous developmental cycle of the human coccidian *Cyclospora cayetanensis*. J. Parasitol. 106 (2), 295–307.

Ghimire, T.R., Bhattarai, N., 2019. A survey of gastrointestinal parasites of goats in a goat market in Kathmandu, Nepal. J. Parasit. Dis. 43 (4), 686–695.

Giangaspero, A., Gasser, R.B., 2019. Human cyclosporiasis. Lancet Infect. Dis. 19 (7), e226–e236.

Graczyk, T.K., Ortega, Y.R., Conn, D.B., 1998. Recovery of waterborne oocysts of *Cyclospora cayetanensis* by Asian freshwater clams (*Corbicula fluminea*). Am. J. Trop. Med. Hyg. 59 (6), 928–932.

Helmy, M.M., 2010. *Cyclospora cayetanensis*: a review, focusing on some of the remaining questions about cyclosporiasis. Infect. Disord. Drug Targets 10 (5), 368–375.

Herwaldt, B.L., 2000. *Cyclospora cayetanensis*: a review, focusing on the outbreaks of cyclospo-riasis in the 1990s. Clin. Infect. Dis. 31 (4), 1040–1057.

Herwaldt, B.L., Ackers, M.L., 1997. An outbreak in 1996 of cyclosporiasis associated with im-ported raspberries. The *Cyclospora* working group. N. Engl. J. Med. 336 (22), 1548–1556.

Hussein, E.M., Abdul-Manaem, A.H., El-Attary, S.L., 2005. *Cyclospora cayetanensis* oocysts in sputum of a patient with active pulmonary tuberculosis, case report in Ismailia, Egypt. J. Egypt. Soc. Parasitol. 35 (3), 787–793.

Insulander, M., Svenungsson, B., Lebbad, M., Karlsson, L., de Jong, B., 2010. A foodborne outbreak of *Cyclospora* infection in Stockholm, Sweden. Foodborne Pathog. Dis. 7 (12), 1585–1587.

Karanja, R.M., Gatei, W., Wamae, N., 2007. Cyclosporiasis: an emerging public health con-cern around the world and in Africa. Afr. Health Sci. 7 (2), 62–67.

Katz, D.E., Taylor, D.N., 2001. Parasitic infections of the gastrointestinal tract. Gastroenterol. Clin. N. Am. 30 (3), 797.

Kłudkowska, M., Pielok, Ł., Frąckowiak, K., Paul, M., 2017. Intestinal coccidian parasites as an underestimated cause of travellers' diarrhoea in Polish immunocompetent patients. Acta Parasitol. 62 (3), 630–638.

Kumar, P., Vats, O., Kumar, D., Singh, S., 2017. Coccidian intestinal parasites among immu-nocompetent children presenting with diarrhea: are we missing them? Trop. Parasitol. 7 (1), 37–40.

Li, G., Xiao, S., Zhou, R., Li, W., Wadeh, H., 2007. Molecular characterization of *Cyclospora*-like organism from dairy cattle. Parasitol. Res. 100 (5), 955–961.

Li, J., Dong, H., Wang, R., Yu, F., Wu, Y., Chang, Y., Wang, C., Qi, M., Zhang, L., 2017. An investigation of parasitic infections and review of molecular characterization of the in-testinal protozoa in nonhuman primates in China from 2009 to 2015. Int. J. Parasitol. Parasites Wildl. 6 (1), 8–15.

Li, J., Cui, Z., Qi, M., Zhang, L., 2020a. Advances in cyclosporiasis diagnosis and therapeutic intervention. Front. Cell. Infect. Microbiol. 10, 43.

Li, J., Wang, R., Chen, Y., Xiao, L., Zhang, L., 2020b. *Cyclospora cayetanensis* infection in hu-mans: biological characteristics, clinical features, epidemiology, detection method and treatment. Parasitology 147 (2), 160–170.

Llanes, R., Velázquez, B., Reyes, Z., Somarriba, L., 2013. Co-infection with *Cyclospora cay-etanensis* and *Salmonella typhi* in a patient with HIV infection and chronic diarrhoea. Pathog. Glob. Health 107 (1), 38–39.

Looney, W.J., 1998. *Cyclospora* species as a cause of diarrhoea in humans. Br. J. Biomed. Sci. 55 (2), 157–161.

Marangi, M., Koehler, A.V., Zanzani, S.A., Manfredi, M.T., Brianti, E., Giangaspero, A., Gasser, R.B., 2015. Detection of *Cyclospora* in captive chimpanzees and macaques by a quantitative PCR-based mutation scanning approach. Parasit. Vectors 8, 274.

Marcos, L.A., Gotuzzo, E., 2013. Intestinal protozoan infections in the immunocompromised host. Curr. Opin. Infect. Dis. 26 (4), 295–301.

Milord, F., Lampron-Goulet, E., St-Amour, M., Levac, E., Ramsay, D., 2012. *Cyclospora caye-tanensis*: a description of clinical aspects of an outbreak in Quebec, Canada. Epidemiol. Infect. 140 (4), 626–632.

Mota, P., Rauch, C.A., Edberg, S.C., 2000. Microsporidia and *Cyclospora*: epidemiology and assessment of risk from the environment. Crit. Rev. Microbiol. 26 (2), 69–90.

Nsagha, D.S., Njunda, A.L., Assob, N.J.C., Ayima, C.W., Tanue, E.A., Kibu, O.D., Kwenti, T.E., 2016. Intestinal parasitic infections in relation to CD4(+) T cell counts and diarrhea in HIV/AIDS patients with or without antiretroviral therapy in Cameroon. BMC Infect. Dis. 16, 9.

Okhuysen, P.C., 2001. Traveler's diarrhea due to intestinal protozoa. Clin. Infect. Dis. 33 (1), 110–114.

Orozco-Mosqueda, G.E., Martínez-Loya, O.A., Ortega, Y.R., 2014. *Cyclospora* cayetanensis in a pediatric hospital in Morelia, México. Am. J. Trop. Med. Hyg. 91 (3), 537–540.

Ortega, Y.R., Sanchez, R., 2010. Update on *Cyclospora cayetanensis*, a food-borne and water-borne parasite. Clin. Microbiol. Rev. 23 (1), 218–234.

Ortega, Y.R., Nagle, R., Gilman, R.H., Watanabe, J., Miyagui, J., Quispe, H., Kanagusuku, P., Roxas, C., Sterling, C.R., 1997. Pathologic and clinical findings in patients with cyclosporiasis and a description of intracellular parasite life-cycle stages. J. Infect. Dis. 176 (6), 1584–1589.

Pons, S., Darles, C., Aguilon, P., Gaillard, T., Brisou, P., 2012. Watery diarrhea in an immune-competent traveler. J. Clin. Microbiol. 50 (12), 3821–4194.

Puente, S., Morente, A., García-Benayas, T., Subirats, M., Gascón, J., González-Lahoz, J.M., 2006. Cyclosporiasis: a point source outbreak acquired in Guatemala. J. Travel Med. 13 (6), 334–337.

Richardson Jr., R.F., Remler, B.F., Katirji, B., Murad, M.H., 1998. Guillain-Barré syndrome after *Cyclospora* infection. Muscle Nerve 21 (5), 669–671.

Shields, J.M., Olson, B.H., 2003. *Cyclospora* cayetanensis: a review of an emerging parasitic coccidian. Int. J. Parasitol. 33 (4), 371–391.

Shlim, D.R., 2002. *Cyclospora cayetanensis*. Clin. Lab. Med. 22 (4), 927–936.

Sifuentes-Osornio, J., Porras-Cortés, G., Bendall, R.P., Morales-Villarreal, F., Reyes-Terán, G., Ruiz-Palacios, G.M., 1995. *Cyclospora* cayetanensis infection in patients with and without AIDS: biliary disease as another clinical manifestation. Clin. Infect. Dis. 21 (5), 1092–1097.

Sloan, V.S., 2001. Reiter syndrome following protracted symptoms of *Cyclospora* infection. Emerg. Infect. Dis. 7 (6), 1070.

Sun, T., Ilardi, C.F., Asnis, D., Bresciani, A.R., Goldenberg, S., Roberts, B., Teichberg, S., 1996. Light and electron microscopic identification of *Cyclospora* species in the small intestine. Evidence of the presence of asexual life cycle in human host. Am. J. Clin. Pathol. 105 (2), 216–220.

Thima, K., Mori, H., Praevanit, R., Mongkhonmu, S., Waikagul, J., Watthanakulpanich, D., 2014. Recovery of *Cyclospora cayetanensis* among asymptomatic rural Thai schoolchildren. Asian Pac. J. Trop. Med. 7 (2), 119–123.

Tiwari, B.R., Ghimire, P., Malla, S., Sharma, B., Karki, S., 2013. Intestinal parasitic infection among the HIV-infected patients in Nepal. J. Infect. Dev. Ctries. 7 (7), 550–555.

Udeh, E.O., Obiezue, R.N.N., Okafor, F.C., Ikele, C.B., Okoye, I.C., Otuu, C.A., 2019. Gastrointestinal parasitic infections and immunological status of HIV/AIDS coinfected individuals in Nigeria. Ann. Glob. Health 85 (1), 99.

Yadav, P., Khalil, S., Mirdha, B.R., 2016. Molecular appraisal of intestinal parasitic infection in transplant recipients. Indian J. Med. Res. 144 (2), 258–263.

Yamada, M., Hatama, S., Ishikawa, Y., Kadota, K., 2014. Intranuclear coccidiosis caused by *Cyclospora* spp. in calves. J. Vet. Diagn. Investig. 26 (5), 678–682.

Zar, F.A., El-Bayoumi, E., Yungbluth, M.M., 2001. Histologic proof of acalculous cholecystitis due to *Cyclospora cayetanensis*. Clin. Infect. Dis. 33 (12), E140–E141.

Zhao, G.H., Cong, M.M., Bian, Q.Q., Cheng, W.Y., Wang, R.J., Qi, M., Zhang, L.X., Lin, Q., Zhu, X.Q., 2013. Molecular characterization of *Cyclospora*-like organisms from golden snub-nosed monkeys in Qinling Mountain in Shaanxi province, northwestern China. PLoS ONE 8 (2), e58216.

Zorbozan, O., Quliyeva, G., Tunalı, V., Özbilgin, A., Turgay, N., Gökengin, A.D., 2018. Intestinal protozoa in HIV-infected patients: a retrospective analysis. Turkiye Parazitol. Derg. 42 (3), 187–190.

CHAPTER 4

Epidemiology in human and animals

Contents

4.1 Introduction

Cyclosporiasis is a gastrointestinal disease caused by the genus *Cyclospora* of an apicomplexan parasite. As of today, 22 valid species of *Cyclospora* have been identified in humans and a number of animals, including vipers, moles, myriapodes, rodents, monkeys, and humans (McAllister et al., 2018; Li et al., 2020). *Cyclospora cayetanensis* is the only documented species in humans (Ortega and Sanchez, 2010; Li et al., 2020) that typically induces periodic profuse watery diarrhea (Shields and Olson, 2003; Ortega and Sanchez, 2010; Almeria et al., 2019; Giangaspero and Gasser, 2019). There have been considerable investigations of *Cyclospora* infections in humans and animals worldwide, especially since the large outbreaks of human cyclosporiasis in North America in the mid-1990s (Almeria et al., 2019; Giangaspero and Gasser, 2019).

Cyclospora and Cyclosporiasis
https://doi.org/10.1016/B978-0-12-821616-3.00003-5

C. cayetanensis infections in humans have been documented in over 56 countries of the world, of which 13 have recorded cyclosporiasis outbreaks (Data updated up to December 2018) (Li et al., 2020), which resulted in significant economic loss and public health concern in the countries. In recent past, large-scale human cyclosporiasis outbreaks have occurred in 2013 and 2018 in multiple states of the United States (Abanyie et al., 2015; Casillas et al., 2018). Current research efforts have also come up with some new *Cyclospora* species in animals, such as *Cyclospora papionis* in the captured baboons in Kenya (Li et al., 2011) and *Cyclospora macacae* in the rhesus monkeys in China (Li et al., 2015).

4.2 *C. cayetanensis* epidemiology in humans

Through epidemiological investigations, *C. cayetanensis* has been reported among humans in more than 56 countries that cover all five human-inhabited continents of the world (Fig. 4.1). A total of 5478 investigation cases and 8367 cases of outbreaks and case reports have been documented in humans globally (Table 4.1).

Among the geographical locations, the Americas and Asia have more detected cases of cyclosporiasis. In Asia, such as Nepal, India, and China reported the maximum number of cases of *C. cayetanensis* infection. In Americas, most of the infections have been documented in the United States, Peru, Canada, Guatemala, and Haiti (Table 4.1).

4.2.1 Outbreaks of human cyclosporiasis

Up to December 2018, at least 13 countries have documented cyclosporiasis outbreaks, involving approximately 6557 human cases. Among these countries, the American and European countries including Peru, Mexico, the United States, Canada, and the United Kingdom have reported the most cases (Table 4.2).

The first recorded outbreak of *C. cayetanensis* (termed as "alga-like organism" at that time) infection occurred among 55 British expatriates with prolonged diarrhea in Nepal, between June and November 1989 (Shlim et al., 1991). The first reported outbreak of diarrheal illness associated with *Cyclospora* infection in the United States can be traced back to 1990 (Huang et al., 1995). Until 1996, more than 1400 cases of cyclosporiasis have been recorded as multistate outbreaks in the United States and Canada (Herwaldt and Ackers, 1997). In the United States, the recent large outbreaks of cyclosporiasis have occurred in 2013 and 2018, including 643 and 761 reported cases, respectively (Abanyie et al., 2015; Casillas et al., 2018).

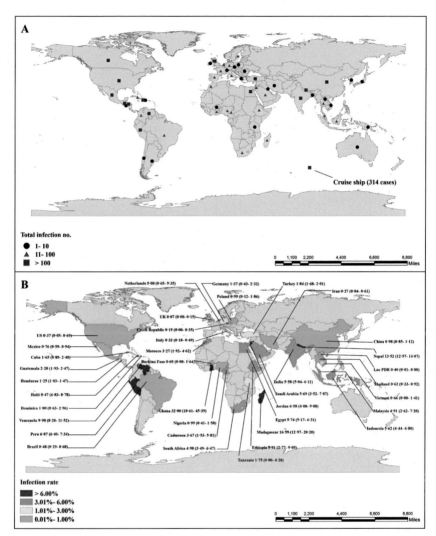

Fig. 4.1 Number of documented human *C. cayetanensis* infections and prevalence worldwide. Number of documented infection cases (A) and prevalence (B) worldwide, and 95% confidence intervals are shown in bracket.

4.2.2 Investigation

Altogether 13,845 cases of *C. cayetanensis* infection have been recorded in humans through epidemiological studies (5478), outbreak investigations (6557), and case reporting (1810) (Tables 4.2–4.4). The overall prevalence of cyclosporiasis among humans is estimated at 3.55% (5478/154,410) in the world. Asia (5.63%, 2771/49,254) and Africa (5.33%, 554/10,401) have shown greater prevalence than the Americas (3.03%, 1625/53,775) and

Table 4.1 Summary of *Cyclospora cayetanensis* infections and cases in humans worldwide.

Country	Sample number	Ratio (%) [95 CI]	Positive cases in investigations	Infection cases (= outbreaks + case reports)	Positive cases in outbreaks	Positive cases in case reports
Asia	**49,254**	**5.63% [5.42–5.83]**	**2771**	**106**	**67**	**39**
Bangladesh	19,412	0.98% [0.85–1.12]	191	6		6 cases
China	1459	5.62% [4.44–6.80]	82	4		4 cases
Indonesia	7082	5.58% [5.04–6.11]	395	5		5 cases
India	1097	0.27% [0.04–0.61]	3	1		1 case
Iran				6		6 cases
Japan	380	6.58% [4.08–9.08]	25	1		1 case
Jordan				6		6 cases
Korea	991	0.40% [0.01–0.80]	4			
Kuwait	346	4.91% [2.62–7.20]	17	1		1 case
Lao PDR	14,856	13.52% [12.97–14.07]	2009	67	67 cases	
Malaysia	439	5.69% [3.52–7.87]	25	3		3 cases
Nepal	2739	0.62% [0.33–0.92]	17	6		6 cases
Papua New Guinea	453	0.66% [0.00–1.41]	3			
Saudi Arabia						
Thailand						
Vietnam						
Europe	**41,186**	**1.28% [1.17–1.39]**	**528**	**497**	**233**	**264**
Czech Republic	3097	0.19% [0.00–0.35]	6	40		40 cases
France				3		3 cases
Ireland	5391	0.33% [0.18–0.49]	18	8		8 cases
Italy	583	1.37% [0.43–2.32]	8	36	34 cases	2 cases
Germany						

Country						
Greece	100	5.00% [0.65–9.35]	5	1		1 case
Netherlands	504	0.99% [0.12–1.86]	5	44	14 cases	30 cases
Poland				3	3 cases	1 case
Romania				1		
Spain				90	7 cases	83 cases
Sweden				18	18 cases	
Switzerland				2		2 cases
Turkey	26,137	1.84% [1.68–2.01]	482	48		48 cases
UK	5374	0.07% [0.00–0.15]	4	203	157 cases	46 cases
Africa	**10,401**	**5.33% [4.89–5.76]**	**554**	**12**	**0**	**566**
Burkina Faso	291	0.69% [0.00–1.64]	2			
Cameroon	300	3.67% [1.53–5.81]	11	1		1 case
Egypt	6411	5.74% [5.17–6.31]	368			
Ethiopia	220	5.91% [2.77–9.05]	13			
Ghana	50	32.00% [18.61–45.39]	16			
Morocco	673	3.27% [1.92–4.62]	22			
Madagascar	410	16.59% [12.97–20.20]	68			
Nigeria	1109	0.99% [0.41–1.58]	11	11		11 cases
South Africa	823	4.98% [3.49–6.47]	41			
Tanzania	114	1.75% [0.00–4.20]	2			
Americas	**53,569**	**3.03% [2.89–3.18]**	**1625**	**7436**	**5943**	**1493**
Argentina	4969			3		3 cases
Brazil		0.48% [0.29–0.68]	24	2		2 cases
Canada				942	941 cases	1 case
Chile				4		4 cases
Colombia				31	31 cases	

Continued

Table 4.1 Summary of *Cyclospora cayetanensis* infections and cases in humans worldwide—cont'd

Country	Sample number	Ratio (%) [95 CI]	Positive cases in investigations	Infection cases (= outbreaks + case reports)	Positive cases in outbreaks	Positive cases in case reports
Cuba	1094	1.65% [0.89–2.40]	18	1		1 case
Dominica	501	1.80% [0.63–2.96]	9			
El Salvador				4	4 cases	
Guatemala	11,340	2.20% [1.93–2.47]	250	1		1 cases
Haiti	2681	8.47% [6.83–8.78]	227	1		1 case
Honduras	9985	1.25% [1.03–1.47]	125	1		
Mexico	9162	0.76% [0.59–0.94]	70	126	101 cases	25 cases
Peru	11,177	6.87% [6.40–7.34]	768	301	127 cases	174 cases
US	1357	0.37% [0.05–0.69]	5	6019	4739 cases	1280 cases
Venezuela	1303	9.90% [8.28–11.52]	129	1		1 case
Oceania				**2**		**2**
Australia				2		2 cases
Cruise ship				314	314 cases	
Total	154,410	3.55% [3.46–3.64]	5478	8367	6557 cases	1810 cases

Table 4.2 Documented outbreaks of *Cyclospora cayetanensis* infection in humans.

Country (site)	Outbreak period	Case numbers	Suspected sources	References
Nepal, Kathmandu	June to November 1989	55 cases	British expatriates	Shlim et al., 1991
US, Illinois	July to August 1990	11 cases	Water services	Huang et al., 1995
Nepal, Pokhara	June 1994	12 cases	River and municipal water	Rabold et al., 1994
US, Florida	June 1995	45 cases	Fresh raspberries and strawberries from Guatemala and Chile	Herwaldt, 2000
US, New York	May to June 1995	32 cases	Food	Herwaldt, 2000
US, multiple states	May to June 1996	1270 cases	Fresh berries	Herwaldt and Ackers, 1997
Canada, two provinces	May to June 1996	195 cases	Fresh berries	Herwaldt and Ackers, 1997
US, cruise ship	March to May 1997	220 cases	Raspberries from Guatemala	CDC, 1997a
US, multistate outbreak	April to June 1997	1012 cases	Fresh raspberries from Guatemala	Herwaldt and Beach, 1999
US, Washington DC	June to July 1997	341 cases	Basil–pesto pasta salad	Herwaldt, 2000
US, Virginia, Maryland, Washington DC	July 1997	48 cases	Basil–pesto pasta salad	CDC, 1997b
US, Virginia	September 1997	21 cases	Fruits	Herwaldt, 2000
US, Florida	December 1997	12 cases	Mesclun salad from Peru	Herwaldt, 2000
US, Georgia	May 1998	17 cases	Fruits salad	Herwaldt, 2000
Canada, Ontario	May 1998	22 cases	Raspberries	CDC, 1998
US, Florida	May 1999	94 cases	Fruits and berry	Herwaldt, 2000
US, Missouri	July 1999	62 cases	Basil imported from Mexico or US	Lopez et al., 2001

Continued

Table 4.2 Documented outbreaks of *Cyclospora cayetanensis* infection in humans—cont'd

Country (site)	Outbreak period	Case numbers	Suspected sources	References
Canada, Ontario	May 1999	104 cases	Berry	Herwaldt, 2000
US, Pennsylvania	June 2000	54 cases	Imported Raspberries	Ho et al., 2002
Mexico	April 2001	101 cases	Attending the same wedding reception	Ayala-Gaytán et al., 2004
Germany	December 2000 to January 2001	34 cases	Salad side dishes from lettuce imported from southern Europe	Döller et al., 2002
Canada, British Columbia	May 2001	17 cases	Basil imported from US	Hoang et al., 2005
Netherlands	September 2001	14 cases	Dutch participants at a scientific meeting in Bogor, Indonesia	Blans et al., 2005
Colombia, Medellín	April 2002	31 cases	Salad and juice	Botero-Garcés et al., 2006
Canada	2003	11 cases	Cilantro	Kozak et al., 2013
Spain	May 2003	7 cases	Traveling to Antigua Guatemala	Puente et al., 2006
US, Pennsylvania	June to July 2004	96 cases	Snow Peas	CDC, 2004
Peru, Lima	November 2004	127 cases	Peruvian naval recruits	Torres-Slimming et al., 2006
Canada	2004 to 2006	17 cases	Either mangoes or basil	Kozak et al., 2013
Canada, Ontario	2005	44 cases	Fresh basil	Kozak et al., 2013
Canada, Quebec	June 2005	200 cases	Basil	Kozak et al., 2013
Canada, Quebec	July to September 2005	142 cases	Food	Milord et al., 2012
Canada, British Columbia	2006	28 cases	Basil or garlic	Kozak et al., 2013
Canada, British Columbia	May to July 2007	29 cases	Strawberries, Romaine lettuce, Garlic, Red peppers, Cilantro, Basil	Shah et al., 2009

Location	Date	Cases	Vehicle	Reference
Sweden, Stockholm	May and June 2009	18 cases	Sugar snap peas from Guatemala	Insulander et al., 2010
Cruise ship: multiple countries	May to June 2010	314 cases	Cruise ship passengers	Gibbs et al., 2013
El Salvador	May to June 2011	4 cases	US military training	Kasper et al., 2012
US, 25 states	June to August 2013	643 cases	Cilantro from Mexico	CDC, 2013
Poland	November 2013	3 cases	Traveling to Indonesia	Bednarska et al., 2015
Canada	June to September 2015	97 cases	Traveling to Mexico	Nichols et al., 2015
UK	June to September 2015	79 cases	Traveling to Mexico	Nichols et al., 2015
Canada, Ontario	fall of 2015	35 cases	Fresh sugar snap peas from Guatemala	Whitfield et al., 2015
UK	July 2017	78 cases	Traveling to Mexico	Marques et al., 2017
USA	May to July 2018	761 cases	Salads and different fresh produce	Casillas et al., 2018
Total		**6557 cases**		

Table 4.3 Epidemiological investigation of *Cyclospora cayetanensis* infection in humans.

Country (site)	Period	Populations	Sample number	Positive number	Prevalence	Detection methods	References
Asia							
China, Anhui	2001	Patients with diarrhea	610	14	2.30%	Auramine–phenol and modified acid-fast stain	Wang et al., 2002
China, Yunnan	June 2007 to October 2009	Patients with diarrhea	378	15	3.97%	Acid-fast satin	Zhang et al., 2002
China, Henan		Hospitalized patients Epidemic features: rainy season	11,554	81	0.70%	Modified acid-fast stain and PCR	Zhou et al., 2011
China, Henan	2011–2015	Hospitalized patients	6579	76	1.16%	PCR	Li et al., 2017a
China, Shanghai	2013	Diarrheal patient Epidemic features: rainy season	291	5	1.72%	PCR	Jiang et al., 2018
Indonesia, Jakarta	January 1995 to July 1998	Gastrointestinal illness or diarrhea of American families	99	9	9.09%		Fryauff et al., 1999
Indonesia, Jakarta	January 1995 to July 1998	Gastrointestinal illness or diarrhea of US Embassy Health Unit	206	28	13.59%		Fryauff et al., 1999
Indonesia, Jakarta	January 1995 to July 1998	Indigenous school children	348	2	0.57%		Fryauff et al., 1999
Indonesia, Jakarta	January 1995 to July 1998	Self-reported Gastrointestinal illness or diarrhea of German embassy personnel	253	29	11.46%		Fryauff et al., 1999

Location	Date	Study population	N	Positive	Prevalence	Method	Reference
Indonesia, West Java	August 2000	Junior high school students	285	2	0.70%	Kato-Katz thick smear	Uga et al., 2002
Indonesia, Jakarta	November 2004 to March 2007	HIV/AIDS patients with chronic diarrhea	268	12	4.48%	Modified acid-fast stain	Kurniawan et al., 2009
India		AIDS patients	334	22	6.59%	Modified acid-fast stain	Deodhar et al., 2000
India		HIV-seropositive patients	120	4	3.33%		Mohandas et al., 2002
India, Chennai		HIV patients with chronic diarrhea	59	1	1.69%	Microscopy	Kumar et al., 2002b
India	May 2000 to January	HIV individuals with chronic diarrhea	152	1	0.66%		Kumar et al., 2002a
India	July 2004 to June 2006	Adults	50	1	2.00%	Wet mount, Kinyoun's modified acid-fast stain and chromotrope 2R stain	Behera et al., 2008
India, Varanasi	January 2006 to October 2007	HIV positive with diarrhea	366	88	24.04%	Modified acid-fast and Modified safranin stain	Tuli et al., 2008
India, Varanasi	January 2006 to October 2007	Patients with diarrhea	200	3	1.50%	Modified acid-fast and Modified safranin stain	Tuli et al., 2008
India		Chronic diarrhea in HIV patients	34	1	2.94%	Microscopy	Gupta et al., 2008

Continued

Table 4.3 Epidemiological investigation of *Cyclospora cayetanensis* infection in humans—cont'd

Country (site)	Period	Populations	Sample number	Positive number	Prevalence	Detection methods	References
India, Pune	March 2002 to March 2007	HIV patients with diarrhea	137	1	0.73%	Microscopy and special stain	Kulkarni et al., 2009
India, Varanasi	January 2006 to December 2008	HIV patients	450	92	20.44%	Modified safranin stain, fluorescence microscopy and PCR	Tuli et al., 2010
India, Varanasi	January 2006 to December 2008	HIV negative patient	200	3	1.50%	Modified safranin stain, fluorescence microscopy and PCR	Tuli et al., 2010
India, Maharashtra	September 2007 to August 2009	Individuals with variable gastrointestinal (GI) symptoms	310	33	10.65%	Modified Ziehl-Neelsen stain	Gupta, 2011
India, Jamnagar	January 2009 to December 2010	HIV patients with diarrhea	544	12	2.21%	Modified Ziehl-Neelsen stain	Mathur et al., 2013
India		HIV patients	242	6	2.48%	Modified Ziehl-Neelsen stain	Ahmed and Chowdhary, 2015
India, Chennai	July to October 2009	Patients	200	1	0.50%	Microscopy	Chopra and Dworkin, 2013

Location	Date	Population	Sample	Positive	Percentage	Method	Reference
India, Chennai	January to June of 2013	Individuals (0–50 years) in low socioeconomic areas	256	57	22.27%	Modified Ziehl-Neelsen stain	Jeevitha et al., 2014
India, Mumbai	February 2006 to April 2008	HIV patients	192	3	1.56%	Light microscopy	Ahmed and Chowdhary, 2013
India	June 2012 to May 2013	Patients with diarrhea	800	19	2.38%	Light microscopy and nested PCR–RFLP	Yadav et al., 2016
India	June 2012 to May 2013	Patients with coinfection of *Entamoeba histolytica*	356	26	7.30%	Microscopy, DNA dot blot and PCR	Nath et al., 2015
India, Pune		HIV patients with diarrhea	45	2	4.44%	Ziehl-Neelsen stain	Shah et al., 2016
India, New Delhi	July 2011 to June 2013	Transplant recipients with diarrhea	38	2	5.26%	Modified Ziehl-Neelsen stain	Yadav et al., 2015
India, New Delhi	December 2015 to May 2016	Children (0–15 years) with diarrhea	200	5	2.50%	Wet mount and modified acid-fast stain	Kumar et al., 2017
India, Chennai	January 2002 to December 2014	HIV patients	829	11	1.33%	Wet mounts and modified acid-fast stain	Swathirajan et al., 2017
India, Rajasthan	September 2014 to April 2016	Patients with diarrhea and other gastrointestinal symptoms	968	1	0.10%	Modified Ziehl-Neelsen stain	Saurabh et al., 2017

Continued

Table 4.3 Epidemiological investigation of *Cyclospora cayetanensis* infection in humans—cont'd

Country (site)	Period	Populations	Sample number	Positive number	Prevalence	Detection methods	References
Iran	May 2010 to May 2011	HIV infected patients with persistent and/or recurrent diarrhea	356	1	0.28%	PCR	Agholi et al., 2013
Iran, Shiraz	October 2009 to October 2014	Immunodeficient patients with recurrent persistent or chronic diarrhea	741	2	0.27%	Microscopy and molecular biological analysis	Agholi et al., 2016
Jordan	September 1999 to September 2001	Patients with gastroenteritis	200	12	6.00%	Fluorescence microscopy and modified acid-fast stain	Nimri, 2003
Jordan, Bedouins		Patients acute or persistent diarrhea	180	13	7.22%	Modified Ziehl-Neelsen stain	Nimri and Meqdam, 2004
Loa PDR	February 2002 to June 2003	Patients with diarrhea	686	1	0.15%	Direct microscopy using ultraviolet and DIC	Kimura et al., 2005
Lao PDR	May 2012	Inhabitants in a village	305	3	0.98%	PCR	Ribas et al., 2017
Malaysia, Kelantan	March 2008 to June 2010	HIV patients	346	17	4.91%	Modified Ziehl-Neelsen acid-fast stain	Asma et al., 2011
Nepal, Kathmandu		Individuals with gastrointestinal symptoms	964	108	11.20%	Standard microbiological and molecular genetic techniques	Hoge et al., 1995

Country	Date period	Population	Total	Positive	Percentage	Method	Reference
Nepal	April to June 1994	Children less than 5 years with diarrhea	124	6	4.84%	Direct microscopy and modified acid-fast stain	Hoge et al., 1995
Nepal	April to June 1994	Children less than 5 years without diarrhea	103	2	1.94%	Direct microscopy and modified acid-fast stain	Hoge et al., 1995
Nepal	April 1995 to November 2000	Expatriate adults with diarrheal symptoms	77	25	32.47%	Direct microscopy and modified acid-fast stain	Shlim et al., 1999
Nepal	April 1995 to November 2000	Symptomatic and asymptomatic patients Epidemic features: summer and rainy season of the year	6562	1619	24.67%	Direct microscopy examination and modified acid-fast stain	Sherchand and Cross, 2001
Nepal	5-year retrospective analysis	Preschool and school-going children	1790	18	1.01%		Easow et al., 2005
Nepal	October 1999 to August 2002	Patients with diarrhea Epidemic features: children aged 10 years and summer (rainy season)	1397	128	9.16%	Direct microscopy using ultraviolet and DIC	Kimura et al., 2005
Nepal, Pokhara	April 1998 to March 2004	Children less than 5 years with persistent diarrhea	253	2	0.79%	Ziehl-Neelsen stain	Mukhopadhyay et al., 2007
Nepal	2006 to 2007	Camps in rural areas	205	7	3.41%	Microscopy	Rai et al., 2008

Continued

Table 4.3 Epidemiological investigation of *Cyclospora cayetanensis* infection in humans—cont'd

Country (site)	Period	Populations	Sample number	Positive number	Prevalence	Detection methods	References
Nepal	October 2007 to September 2008	Pediatric patients	863	2	0.23%	Modified Ziehl-Neelsen stain	Amatya et al., 2011
Nepal	March 2001 to 2003	Visitors (over 18 years)	381	31	8.14%	Microbiological assay, PCR and enzyme immunoassay	Pandey et al., 2011
Nepal	March 2005 to December 2008	HIV infected people	167	14	8.38%	Microscopy examination	Tiwari et al., 2013
Nepal, Lalitpur	July to December 2011	School children	1392	23	1.65%	Modified Ziehl-Neelsen stain	Tandukar et al., 2013
Nepal, Kathmandu	May to November 2014	School children (3–14 years) Epidemic features: peaking at 3–5 year age group with diarrheal symptoms; rainy season (June–August); household keeping livestock and consumers of raw vegetables/fruits	507	20	3.94%	Modified Kinyoun acid-fast stain	Bhandari et al., 2015

Location	Date	Population	n	Positive	%	Method	Reference
Nepal, Kathmandu	November 2013	A slum in a valley Epidemic features: drinking water	71	4	5.63%	Modified Ziehl-Neelsen acid-fast stain	Bhattachan et al., 2017
Saudi Arabia, Jeddah	March to May 2000	Children (<5 years) with diarrheal disease	63	7	11.11%	Staining	Al-Braiken et al., 2003
Saudi Arabia, Jeddah	March to May 2000	Asymptomatic children (<5 years)	190	8	4.21%	Staining	Al-Braiken et al., 2003
Saudi Arabia, Riyadh		Immunocompromised patients	136	8	5.88%	Modified Ziehl-Neelsen and modified trichrome stains	Al-Megrin, 2010
Saudi Arabia, Taif		Chronic renal failure (CRF) patients	50	2	4.00%	Dodified Ziehl-Neelsen stain	Hawash et al., 2015
Thailand		AIDS patients with diarrhea	45	1	2.22%	Staining	Manatsathit et al., 1996
Thailand		HIV patients	64	3	4.69%	Staining	Viriyavejakul et al., 2009
Thailand, Lopburi	2005	HIV/AIDS patients	90	1	1.11%	Modified Ziehl-Neelsen satin	Saksirisampant et al., 2009
Thailand		Rural villagers individuals Epidemic features: school children aged 5–12 years	2540	12	0.47%	Modified acid-fast stain and PCR	Thima et al., 2014

Continued

Table 4.3 Epidemiological investigation of *Cyclospora cayetanensis* infection in humans—cont'd

Country (site)	Period	Populations	Sample number	Positive number	Prevalence	Detection methods	References
Vietnam, Hanam	July to October 2008 and April to June 2009	Household individuals	453	3	0.66%	Microscopy examination	Pham-Duc et al., 2013
Europe							
Czech Republic	February 2009 to March 2010	Patients Epidemic features: travel from the endemic countries	3097	6	0.19%	Standard parasitological methods	Jelínková et al., 2011
Italy, Rome	May 2006 to December 2008	Patients	5351	7	0.13%	Modified Ziehl-Neelsen acid-fast stain, and PCR	Masucci et al., 2011
Italy, Apulia	Spring 2012 to Winter 2014	Human	40	11	27.50%	qPCR–SSCP	Giangaspero et al., 2015
Germany	May to September 1995	Patients returning from developing countries with diarrhea	469	5	1.07%	Acid-fast stain	Jelinek et al., 1997
Germany, Munich	August 2006 to November 2009	Travelers returning from the tropics with diarrhea	114	3	2.63%	PCR	Paschke et al., 2011
Netherlands	February to April 2001	Travelers returning from tropics and subtropics with diarrhea	100	5	5.00%	qRT-PCR	Varma et al., 2003

Country	Time period	Population	Sample	Positive	Percentage	Method	Reference
Poland	June 2013 to January 2017	Travelers returning from hot climates got hospitalized due to diarrhea and other gastrointestinal symptoms Epidemic features: international travels, particularly to developing countries with lower economic and sanitary conditions	221	3	1.36%	acid-fast stain	Khudkowska et al., 2017
Poland	2007–2015	Immunocompetent patients	46	1	2.17%	Ziehl-Neelsen stain and PCR	Bednarska et al., 2018
Poland	2007–2015	Immunocompromised patients	237	1	0.42%	Ziehl-Neelsen stain and PCR	Bednarska et al., 2018
Turkey, Izmir	October 2003 to October 2004	Patients with gastrointestinal symptoms	4660	23	0.49%	Trichrome stain, and modified Kinyoun's acid-fast stain	Turgay et al., 2012
Turkey, Izmir	June 2004 to June 2005	Patients with diarrhea	554	2	0.36%	Kinyoun acid-fast stain	Aksoy et al., 2014
Turkey	January to December 2005	Outpatients	3925	75	1.91%	Kinyoun's acid-fast stain	Değirmenci et al., 2007

Continued

Table 4.3 Epidemiological investigation of *Cyclospora cayetanensis* infection in humans—cont'd

Country (site)	Period	Populations	Sample number	Positive number	Prevalence	Detection methods	References
Turkey, Kars	March to June 2007	Children (2–6 year)	138	1	0.72%	Modified acid–fast satin	Arslan et al., 2008
Turkey, Istanbul	Summers of 2006 to 2009	Hospitalized patients Epidemic features: 15 were clustered during about 15 days (dry and warm summer)	1876	20	1.07%	Light and epifluorescence microscopy, Kinyoun's modified acid–fast stain, and PCR identify	Ozdamar et al., 2010
Turkey	2009	Patients	6267	7	0.11%	Modified acid–fast stain	Yilmaz et al., 2012
Turkey	May 2009 to April 2010	Patients	5073	187	3.69%	Modified kinyoun's acid–fast satin	Turgay et al., 2007
Turkey		Children with diarrhea	225	1	0.44%	Modified Ehrlich Ziehl-Neelsen satin	Doğan et al., 2012
Turkey, Izmir	September 2005 to April 2006	Individuals in city center and counties Epidemic features: Lower socioeconomic conditions, lack of health insurance, consumption of tap water, eating in common places	873	26	2.98%	Kinyoun acid–fast stain	Erdogan et al., 2012

Location	Period	Population	Total	Positive	Percentage	Method	Reference
Turkey, Malatya	**2006**	Patients with digestive disorder / Epidemic features: immunosuppressed patients	2281	129	5.66%	UV fluorescence and acid-fast stain	Karaman et al., 2015
Turkey		Patients with AIDS	115	3	2.61%	Modified Ziehl-Neelsen satin, and PCR identify	Uysal et al., 2017
Turkey	**April to December 2016**	Patients in Child Intensive Care Unit	150	8	5.33%	Native-Lugol sedimentation and acid fast satin	Birdal Akış and Beyhan, 2018
UK	**October 1993 to September 1994**	Hospitalized patients	5374	4	0.07%	Modified Ziehl-Neelsen satin	Clarke and McIntyre, 1996
Africa							
Burkina Faso, Bobo-Dioulasso	**April to August 2012**	Patients	291	2	0.69%	Modified Ziehl-Neelsen stain	Sangaré et al., 2015
Cameroon	**April to July 2014**	HIV patients without antiretroviral therapy	52	9	17.31%	Modified Ziehl-Neelsen stain	Nsagha et al., 2016
Cameroon	**April to July 2014**	HIV patients with antiretroviral therapy	248	2	0.81%	Modified Ziehl-Neelsen stain	Nsagha et al., 2016
Egypt					1.80%	Modified Ziehl-Neelsen stain	El Naga et al., 1998

Continued

Table 4.3 Epidemiological investigation of *Cyclospora cayetanensis* infection in humans—cont'd

Country (site)	Period	Populations	Sample number	Positive number	Prevalence	Detection methods	References
Egypt		Patients with prolonged watery diarrhea	130	12	9.23%	Modified Ziehl-Neelsen and aniline carbol methyl violet stain	Nassef et al., 1998
Egypt	1998	Patients with diarrhea	300	12	4.00%	Modified Ziehl-Neelsen and Kinyoun acid-fast satin	El Naggar et al., 1999
Egypt		Children with watery diarrhea and protein energy malnutrition (PEM)	155	2	1.29%	Modified Ziehl-Neelsen satin	Osman et al., 1999
Egypt		Immunocompromised patients	150	6	4.00%	Modified Ziehl-Neelsen satin	Abou el Naga, 1999
Egypt, Dakahlia		Patients	3180	134	4.21%	Modified Kinyoun's acid-fast stain	El Shazly et al., 2006
Egypt		Patients receiving chemotherapy			6.30%		Rezk et al., 2001
Egypt		Malnourished children	36	2	5.56%		Rizk and Soliman, 2001
Egypt, Dakahlia		Healthy control children	36	1	2.78%		Rizk and Soliman, 2001

Country	Population	No. examined	No. positive	Prevalence	Method	Reference
Egypt	Immunocompromised patients with severe diarrhea	49	9	18.37%	Microscopy and nested PCR	Helmy et al., 2006
Egypt	Patients with CRF	120	9	7.50%	Modified Ziehl-Neelsen satin	Ali et al., 2000
Egypt	Children with gastro-intestinal symptoms	169	25	14.79%	Modified Ziehl-Neelsen, flow cytometry and RT-qPCR	Hussein, 2007
Egypt	Children without gastrointestinal symptom	350	10	2.86%	Modified Ziehl-Neelsen, flow cytometry and RT-qPCR	Hussein et al., 2007
Egypt, Ismailia	Diarrheic children	140	35	25.00%	Modified Kinyoun stain, auto-fluorescent, oocysts sporulation, and nested PCR	Hussein et al., 2007
Egypt	Immunocompromised patients	100	3	3.00%	Microscopy	Baiomy et al., 2010
Egypt, Minia	Pediatric inpatients and outpatients Immunosuppressed	200	13	6.50%	Modified Ziehl-Neelsen stain	Abdel-Hafeez et al., 2012
Egypt, Minia	Pediatric inpatients and outpatients Immunocompetent	250	3	1.20%	Modified Ziehl-Neelsen stain	Abdel-Hafeez et al., 2012

Continued

Table 4.3 Epidemiological investigation of *Cyclospora cayetanensis* infection in humans—cont'd

Country (site)	Period	Populations	Sample number	Positive number	Prevalence	Detection methods	References
Egypt, Alexandria	December 2012 to November 2013	Mentally handicapped individuals	200	15	7.50%	Modified acid-fast stain	Shehata and Hassanein, 2015
Egypt, Alexandria	January to April 2013	Municipality solid waste workers	346	7	2.02%	Modified Ziehl-Neelsen satin	Eassa et al., 2016
Egypt, Ismailia	May 2012 to September 2014	Cyclosporiasis suspected patients	500	70	14.00%	Both staining and autofluorescence and Real-time PCR/HRM	Kitajima et al., 2014
Ethiopia, Arba Minch	March to May 2016	ART patients	220	13	5.91%	Sedimentation and modified Ziehl-Neelsen stain	Alemu et al., 2018
Ghana		HIV/AIDS patients with diarrhea	50	16	32.00%	Modified Ziehl-Neelsen and acid fast stain	Opoku et al., 2018
Morocco, Tetouan	May 2012 to June 2013	Schools children (5–14 years)	673	22	3.27%	Ziehl-Neelsen satin	El Fatni et al., 2014
Madagascar, Ambositra	March 2012	School children (4–18 years)	410	68	16.59%	Multiplex real-time PCR	Frickmann et al., 2015
Nigeria, Lagos	March 1999 to April 2000	Outpatients Epidemic features: diarrhea and HIV	1109	11	0.99%	modified Kinyoun carbolfuchsin stain	Alakpa et al., 2002
South Africa	October 2003 to April 2005	Hospitalized attender	528	38	7.20%	Modified Ziehl-Neelson stain	Samie et al., 2009

Location	Date	Population	n	Positive	%	Staining method	Reference
South Africa	October 2003 to April 2005	School children	295	3	1.02%	Modified Ziehl-Neelson stain	Samie et al., 2009
Tanzania		Adults with AIDS-associated diarrhea	59	1	1.69%	Acid-fast stain	Cegielski et al., 1999
Tanzania		Children with chronic diarrhea	55	1	1.82%	Acid-fast stain	Cegielski et al., 1999
Americas							
Brazil, São Paulo	April 1996 to January 2002	Hospitalized patients	4869	14	0.29%	Kinyoun's modified stain	Gonçalves et al., 2005
Brazil	August 2006	Community Individuals	83	9	10.84%	Modifed detergent Ziehl-Neelsen stain	Borges et al., 2009
Brazil, São Paulo	March to September 2013	HIV infected children	17	1	5.88%	Modified Ziehl-Neelsen stain	Fregonesi et al., 2015
Cuba	September 1994 to January 1995	AIDS patients	67	2	2.99%	Direct wet mount and modified Ziehl-Neelsen stain	Escobedo and Núñez, 1999
Cuba, Havana	November 1998	Children (1–5 years)	456	7	1.54%		Mendoza et al., 2001
Cuba, Havana	May to August 1999	Patients with diarrhea	113	5	4.42%	Modified Ziehl-Neelsen stain	Núñez et al., 2003b
Cuba, Habana	May to June 1999	Children in the Pediatric hospital	288	0	0	Ziehl-Neelsen stain	Núñez et al., 2003a
Cuba	July 2000	HIV patients	170	4	2.35%		de de Paz et al., 2003

Continued

Table 4.3 Epidemiological investigation of *Cyclospora cayetanensis* infection in humans—cont'd

Country (site)	Period	Populations	Sample number	Positive number	Prevalence	Detection methods	References
Dominica Republic		Humans	501	9	1.80%	qPCR–MCA	Lalonde et al., 2013
Guatemala	April 1997 to March 1998	Outpatients Epidemic features: most common among children with 1.5 to 9 years old, and persons with gastroenteritis	5552	126	2.27%	Modified acid-fast stain and UV epifluorescence	Bern et al., 1999
Guatemala	April 1997 to March 1998	Outpatients	5520	117	2.12%	Acid-fast stain	Bern et al., 2000
Guatemala	April 1999 to April 2000	Malnourished children	111	1	0.90%	Modified acid-fast stain and epifluorescence	Pratdesaba et al., 2001
Guatemala	April 1999 to April 2000	HIV/AIDS patients	157	6	3.82%	Modified acid-fast stain and epifluorescence	Pratdesaba et al., 2001
Haiti	1990 to 1993	HIV patients with chronic or intermittent diarrhea	804	88	10.95%	Acid-fast stain	Pape et al., 1994
Haiti	January 1997 through January 1998	Local resident	741	59	7.96%	UV fluorescent microscopy, acid-fast or hot safranin stain and sporulated confirm	Eberhard et al., 1999

Location	Date	Population	n	Positive	%	Method	Reference
Haiti	February and April 2001	Children (<10 years)	519	24	4.62%	UV fluorescence	Lopez et al., 2003
Haiti, Portau Prince	???	HIV infected patients and family members	213	1	0.47%	Modified Ziehl-Neelsen stain	Raccurt et al., 2006
Haiti, Portau Prince	January 1997 to August 1998	HIV-infected patients with chronic diarrhea	42	20	47.62%	Acid-fast stain	Verdier et al., 2000
Haiti, Portau Prince	March to September 2007	Chronic diarrhea in HIV patients	74	27	36.49%	PCR	Raccurt et al., 2008
Haiti, Virginia	March 2003 to April 2004	HIV patients with antiretroviral therapy	288	8	2.78%	Modified Kinyoun acid-fast stain	Dillingham et al., 2009
Honduras	2002 to 2011	Hospitalized patients Epidemic features: stool were diarrheic or liquid; children 10 years old or less, Marked seasonality: rainy months	9985	125	1.25%	Ziehl–Neelsen carbolfuchsin satin	Kaminsky et al., 2016
Mexico	March 1997 to January 1998	Children (2–14 years)	272	8	2.94%	Acid-fast Kinyoun stain	Diaz et al., 2003
Mexico		Pediatric patients with leukemia or lymphoma Epidemic features: with diarrhea	13	2	15.38%	Modified Ziehl-Neelsen stain	Jiménez-González et al., 2012

Continued

Table 4.3 Epidemiological investigation of *Cyclospora cayetanensis* infection in humans—cont'd

Country (site)	Period	Populations	Sample number	Positive number	Prevalence	Detection methods	References
Mexico, Michoacan	January 2000 to December 2009	Children (less than 15 years) Epidemic features: rainy season (June–August)	8877	60	0.68%	PCR	Orozco-Mosqueda et al., 2014
Peru	1996 to 1997	Children	5836	63	1.08%	Modified acid-fast stain and autofluorescence microscopy	Madico et al., 1997
Peru, Lima		Dwellers of marginal urban settlements Epidemic features: contamination source appears to be the water	291	121	41.58%	Staining	Burstein Alva, 2005
Peru, Lima		Asymptomatic patients Epidemic features: contamination source appears to be the water	2968	217	7.31%	Staining	Burstein Alva, 2005
Peru, Trujillo	January to December 2004	Children	489	64	13.09%	Ziehl–Neelsen stain	Cordova Paz Soldan et al., 2006

Location	Period	Population	N	Positive	Prevalence	Method	Reference
Peru, Trujillo	January to December 2005	Children (1 month to 9 years)	845	22	2.60%	Ziehl-Neelsen satin	Peréz Cordón et al., 2008
Peru, Cajamarca	June to October 2005	Adult subjects	256	11	4.30%	dot-ELISA	Roldán et al., 2009
Peru	December 2001 to June 2006	Low-income community participants	492	270	54.88%	direct wet mounts and autofluorescence confirm	Nundy et al., 2011
US, Massachusetts	May to November 1993	Patients with diarrhea	1042	3	0.29%	Wet mount, acid-fast stain, modified Kinyoun stain	Ooi et al., 1995
US, Kentucky	March to September 2001	Patients with diarrhea	315	2	0.63%	Kinyoun modified acid-fast stain	Ribes et al., 2004
Venezuela	January 1992 to February 1994	AIDS patients	71	7	9.86%	Modified Ziehl-Neelsen stain	Chacín-Bonilla et al., 2001
Venezuela	January 1992 to February 1994	Children with diarrhea	132	7	5.30%	Modified Ziehl-Neelsen stain	Chacín-Bonilla et al., 2001
Venezuela		Community individuals	212	13	6.13%	Modified Ziehl-Neelsen stain	Chacín-Bonilla et al., 2003
Venezuela, Bolivar	July 2003 to April 2004	Indigenous people	160	19	11.88%	Kinyoun stain	Devera et al., 2005

Continued

Table 4.3 Epidemiological investigation of *Cyclospora cayetanensis* infection in humans—cont'd

Country (site)	Period	Populations	Sample number	Positive number	Prevalence	Detection methods	References
Venezuela, San Carlos Island	August to September 2003	Community individuals Epidemic features: contact with soil contaminated with human feces	515	43	8.35%	Modified Ziehl-Neelsen carbolfuchsin stain	Chacín-Bonilla et al., 2007
Venezuela, Falcon	June to October 2011	Individuals	157	38	24.20%	Direct smear and Kinyoun stain	Cazorla et al., 2012
Venezuela, Maracaibo	September 2008 to October 2007	Patients with HIV/AIDS	56	2	3.57%	Kinyoun coloration and fast Gram-Chromotrope coloration	Rivero-Rodríguez et al., 2013
Total			**154,410**	**5478**	**3.55%**		

Table 4.4 Summary of cyclosporiasis case reports in humans.

Country (site)	Period	Gender	Age	Population	Number of cases	Detection method	References
Asia							
Bangladesh				Indigenous people with diarrhea	6 cases	Modified acid-fast stain	Albert et al., 1994
China				A patient with mixed infection with other coccidian parasites	1 case		Zhang, 2000
China		Male	39-year	A patient having the history of biking trip from Tibet to Nepal	1 case		Dekker and Kager, 2002.
China				A patient with chronic diarrhea, hypoproteinemia and coinfection with *Cryptosporidium parvum*	1 case		Zeng et al., 2005
China, Hong Kong		Female	38-year	HIV patient	1 case	Modified Ziehl-Neelsen acid-fast stain and histological examination	Tsang et al., 2013
India				An acute myeloid leukemia patient	1 case		Jayshree et al., 1998
India				An immunocompromised patient with chronic diarrhea	1 case		Parija et al., 2000

Continued

Table 4.4 Summary of cyclosporiasis case reports in humans—cont'd

Country (site)	Period	Gender	Age	Population	Number of cases	Detection method	References
India				AIDS patient	1 case		Chakrabarti et al., 2004
India			7-month	Infant with incessant crying and refusal of feeds	1 case	Modified Ziehl-Neelsen stain	Iyer, 2006
India, Tamil Nadu	March 2012	Male		An old man with history of watery stool	1 case	Microscopic examination of saline wet smear	Swarna et al., 2013
Iran, Tehran	2014	Female	25-year	HIV patient with symptoms of faintness and fatigue	1 case	Modified acid-fast stain and light and immunofluorescence microscopy	Khanaliha et al., 2015
Japan	1996 to 2001			Three overseas travelers, and one HIV patient	4 cases		Masuda et al., 2002
Japan		Male	42-year	A French man visited Vietnam	1 case	Smear using UV fluorescence microscopy	Naito et al., 2009
Japan		Female	42-year	Resided in Indonesia	1 case	Modified acid fast stain	Sakakibara et al., 2010
Korea	December 2003	Female	14-year	A traveler returning from Indonesia with diarrhea	1 case	Modified acid fast stain	Yu and Sohn, 2003
Kuwait				Indian migrants and local people without history of traveling abroad	6 cases	Modified acid-fast stain and UV fluorescence microscopy	Iqbal et al., 2011

Location	Date	Sex	Age	Patient description	Cases	Stain	Reference
Malaysia				Diarrhea patient	1 case		Sinniah et al., 1994
Papua New Guinea		Male		Diarrhea patients	3 cases		Ashford, 1979
Thailand				A HIV patient	1 case		Wanachiwanawin et al., 1995
Thailand				A patient with coinfection with microsporidium	1 case		Morakote et al., 1995
Thailand			3–year	Malnourished orphan with fever, abdominal distension and relapsing diarrhea	1 case	Modified acid-fast stain	Chokephaibulkit et al., 2001
Thailand	1999 to 2000			Two HIV patients and one patient with prolonged diarrhea	3 cases		Siripanth et al., 2002
Americas							
Argentina	February 1998	Male	60–year	A patient with pulmonary tuberculosis[a] in the respiratory system	1 case	Ziehl–Neelsen stain	Di Gliullo et al., 2000
Argentina				HIV patients with chronic diarrhea	2 cases	Modified acid-fast or safranin stain	Velásquez et al., 2004
Brazil				Asymptomatic patient infected with HIV and HTLV-1	1 case		Schubach et al., 1997
Brazil, São Paulo				A patient	1 case	Modified Kinyoun stain	Fernandes et al., 1998

Continued

Table 4.4 Summary of cyclosporiasis case reports in humans—cont'd

Country (site)	Period	Gender	Age	Population	Number of cases	Detection method	References
Chile		Female	50–year	A patient with explosive diarrhea and weight loss, and the history of visiting to Cuba	1 case		Madrid et al., 1998
Chile				Three patients who traveled to Peru	3 cases	Ziehl–Neelsen stain	Weitz et al., 2009
Cuba					1 case		Núñez Fernández et al., 1995
Canada							Purych et al., 1995
Haiti		Male	45–year	HIV patient with fever, abdominal cramping, chronic diarrhea, and weight loss	1 case	Modified Ziehl–Neelsen stain and histological examination	Llanes et al., 2013
Honduras		Male	33–year	A patient	1 case	Modified Ziehl–Neelsen stain	de Górgolas et al., 2001
Mexico				12 patients (7 had AIDS)	12 cases	Acid–fast stain	Sifuentes–Osornio et al., 1995
Mexico				Children	2 cases	Ziehl–Neelsen stain	Ponce–Macotela et al., 1996
Mexio				Pediatric patients	10 cases	Modified Zehl–Nielsen stain	Vásquez et al., 1998
Mexico		Male	26–year	Airline pilot with episodes of diarrhea after a five-day stay in Lima, Peru	1 case	Ziehl–Neelsen stain	Sánchez–Vega et al., 2014

Location	Date	Gender	Age	Description	Cases	Method	Reference
Peru, Lima	February 1995 to December 1998			Children Epidemic features: warm season (December to May)	174 cases	Ziehl-Neelsen acid-fast stain	Bern et al., 2002
US				Patients having the history of visiting to either Mexico or Thailand	5 cases		Berlin et al., 1994
US				Guillain–Barré syndrome patient with diarrhea	1 case		Richardson Jr. et al., 1998
US	1997 to 2008			FoodNet surveillance data	1110 cases	laboratory-confirm	Hall et al., 2011
US, New York	November 2009	Male	55-year	A kidney transplant recipient from the Dominican Republic living in New York	1 case	Bright fluorescence microscopy	Visvesvara et al., 2013
USA	2018			FoodNet sites surveillance data	163 cases		Marder Mph et al., 2018
Venezuela				A patient with Diarrhea	1 cases		Marín-Leonett et al., 2007
Europe							
France	1995 to 1996			Travelers	11 cases		Junod et al., 1994
France				A HIV patient	1 case		Raguin et al., 1995
Franch				Patients	19 cases		Deluol and Junod, 1996

Continued

Table 4.4 Summary of cyclosporiasis case reports in humans—cont'd

Country (site)	Period	Gender	Age	Population	Number of cases	Detection method	References
France				An AIDS patient having coinfection with *Cryptosporidium* sp.	1 case		Bellagra et al., 1998
France				A tourist back from Dominican Republic	1 case		Estran et al., 2004
France			24–67 years	People complained of diarrhea and weight loss, after a travel abroad	6 cases		Bourée et al., 2007
France		Male	43–year	A traveler stayed in Southeast Asia, including China	1 case	Modified Ziehl–Neelsen acid-fast stain, UV fluorescence microscope	Pons et al., 2012
Germany		Female	70–year	A patient with severe and prolonged diarrhea after a vacation in Singapore, Java and Bali	1 case	Modified Ziehl–Neelsen stain	Petry et al., 1997
Germany		Female	58–year	A patient with severe and prolonged diarrhea after a vacation in Singapore, Java, and Bali	1 case	Modified Ziehl–Neelsen stain	Petry et al., 1997
Greece	July 2000	Male	44–year	A Greek who lived in Germany	1 case	Acid fast stain	Kansouzidou et al., 2004

Country	Date	Sex	Age	Description	Cases	Method	Reference
Ireland				Travelers returned from Nepal and Pakistan	3 cases		220
Italy				AIDS patient	1 case		Crowley et al., 1996
Italy				AIDS patients	2 cases		Maggi et al., 1995
Italy	August 1994	Male	37-year	A traveler returned from Nepal	1 case		Caramello et al., 1995
Italy	October 1994	Female	38-year	Travelers returned from Indonesia	2 cases		Caramello et al., 1995
Italy	August 1997	Male	32-year	A traveler returned from Bolivia and Peru	1 case	UV fluorescence microscope	Drenaggi et al., 1998
Italy	March 2007	Female	63-year	A local patient	1 case	Microscopy detected and PCR	Masucci et al., 2008
Netherlands, Amsterdam	1992 to 1995			Patients	28 cases		van Gool and Dankert, 1996
Netherlands, Amsterdam		Female	60-year	A traveler Returned from Indonesia with persisting diarrhea	1 case		Lammers et al., 1996
Netherlands, Amsterdam		Male	58-year	A person with persisting diarrhea whose wife returned from Indonesia	1 case		Lammers et al., 1996
Romania				A child with acute diarrhea	1 case	Acid-fast stain	Popovici et al., 2003
Spain				Travelers	20 cases		Gascón et al., 1995

Continued

Table 4.4 Summary of cyclosporiasis case reports in humans—cont'd

Country (site)	Period	Gender	Age	Population	Number of cases	Detection method	References
Spain				Travelers to tropical and temperate areas	55 cases		Gascón et al., 2001
Spain				Spanish travelers	7 cases		Ramírez–Olivencia et al., 2008
Spain					1 case		Portillo et al., 2010
Switzerland	May 1999	Male	40–year	A traveler with diarrhea	1 case	Acid-fast stain	Egloff et al., 2001
				HIV-1 patient, traveling to Thailand			
Switzerland, Bern			46–year	A HIV-1 patient Epidemic features: travel to southeast Asia	1 case		Mosimann et al., 1999
Turkey		Male	52–year	Idiopathic hepatic cirrhosis patient with diarrhea and weakness	1 case	Autofluorescent, modified Kinyoun's acid-fast stain	Yazar et al., 2002
Turkey	December 1996	Female	50–year	AIDS patient	1 case	Microscopical analysis	Yazar et al., 2004
Turkey	2000	Male	40–year	AIDS patient	1 case	Kinyoun's acid-fast stain	Yazar et al., 2004
Turkey	2000	Male	7–year	Patient with acute myeloblastic leukemia (AML)	1 case	Acid-fast stain	Yazar et al., 2004
Turkey	2001	Male	52–year	Patient with idiopathic hepatic cirrhosis	1 case	Modified Kinyoun's acid-fast stain and fluorescent microscope	Yazar et al., 2004
Turkey	2002	Female	30–year	Patient with diarrhea	1 case	Modified Kinyoun's acid-fast stain	Yazar et al., 2004

Location	Date	Sex	Age	Clinical presentation	Cases	Staining method	Reference
Turkey	2002	Male	62-year	Patient with diarrhea	1 case	Acid–fast stain	Yazar et al., 2004
Turkey	July 2002	Female	30-year	A patient	1 case	Modified Kinyoun's acid-fast stain	Türk et al., 2004
Turkey, Ankara	August 2003	Female	24-year	Patient with prolonged diarrhea	1 case	Modified acid-fast stain	Koru et al., 2006
Turkey		Male	64-year	Persistent diarrhea, abdominal pain, nausea and vomiting after visiting the Greek Islands	1 case	Kinyoun's modified acid fast stain	Turgay et al., 2006
Turkey	August 2004	Female	67-year	Patients with watery diarrhea	5 cases	Modified acid-fast stain	Sancak et al., 2006
Turkey	August 2004	Female	28-year	Patients with watery diarrhea	5 cases	Modified acid-fast stain	Sancak et al., 2006
Turkey	August 2004	Male	44-year	Patients with watery diarrhea	5 cases	Modified acid-fast stain	Sancak et al., 2006
Turkey	August 2004	Female	27-year	Patients with watery diarrhea and malaise	5 cases	Modified acid-fast stain	Sancak et al., 2006
Turkey	August 2004	Male	31-year	Patients with weight loss, cramping abdominal pain and malaise	5 cases	Modified acid-fast stain	Sancak et al., 2006
Turkey	September 2005			A patient with coinfection with Cryptosporidium	1 case		Aksoy et al., 2007
Turkey, Kayseri		Female	18-year	A patient with diarrhea	1 case	Kinyoun's acid-fast stain	Yazar et al., 2009

Continued

Table 4.4 Summary of cyclosporiasis case reports in humans—cont'd

Country (site)	Period	Gender	Age	Population	Number of cases	Detection method	References
Turkey, Kayseri		Female	26–year	A patient with diarrhea	1 case	Kinyoun's acid-fast stain	Yazar et al., 2009
Turkey, Kayseri		Female	34–year	A patient with diarrhea	1 case	Kinyoun's acid-fast stain	Yazar et al., 2009
Turkey	July 2009			Patients with diarrhea and abdominal pain	2 cases	Direct smear and modified acid-fast stain	Ciçek et al., 2011
Turkey, Van				Local residents without history of travel	7 cases	Formalin–ethyl acetate and modified acid-fast stain	Taş Cengiz et al., 2016
UK	June 1996	Male	74–year	Returning from the Dominican Republic	1 case		Green et al., 2000
UK	June 1996	Female	72–year	An woman whose husband had *Cyclospora* infection	1 case		Green et al., 2000
UK, Scotland	1993 to 2002			Different individuals	42 cases		Stewart et al., 2005
UK		Male	43–year	A patient with fever and diarrhea	1 case		Burrell et al., 2007
UK	2009		59–year	A professor attended the annual digestive diseases meeting in Chicago	1 case	direct smear, UV epifluorescence, and histological examination	Marek et al., 2012

Africa

Location	Date	Sex	Age	Details	Cases	Method	Reference
Egypt, Ismailia		Male	45-year	A patient with active pulmonary tuberculosis (Purulent sputum specimen tested)	1 case	Ziehl–Neelsen stain and PCR	Hussein et al., 2005
Nigeria, Lagos	March 1999 to April 2000			Hospitalized patients Epidemic features: vegetables and water as possible vehicle	11 cases		Alakpa et al., 2003

Oceania

Location	Date	Sex	Age	Details	Cases	Method	Reference
Australia		Female	42-year	A traveler returned from Bali, Indonesia	1 case	Ziehl–Neelsen stain	Butcher et al., 1994
Australia		Female	56-year	A traveler returned from Indonesia	1 case		Pingé–Suttor et al., 2004
Total					**1810 cases**		

[a] Found in sputum sample which is the first instance of the parasite.

Europe (1.28%, 528/41,186). A high prevalence and large number of cases of *C. cayetanensis* have been recorded in Nepal (13.68%) and India (5.58%) in Asia; Madagascar (16.59%) and Egypt (5.74%) in Africa; and Venezuela (9.90%), Peru (6.87%), and Haiti (8.47%) in the Americas.

4.2.3 Case reports

There have been many cases of *C. cayetanensis* infections in humans that are documented as sporadic cases (case reports) globally (Table 4.4). Among the 1810 case reports, a maximum of 1493 cases were reported from the American countries alone and a minimum of 2 cases were observed in Australia.

4.3 Susceptible populations and risk factors

C. cayetanensis infection in humans is associated with several risk factors such as immune status, gastrointestinal diseases, age, hygiene, and sanitary conditions.

4.3.1 Human immune state

C. cayetanensis is among the important opportunistic protozoans of humans (Wiwanitkit, 2006). Host immunodeficiency and diarrhea are two major risk factors that might facilitate the infection of *C. cayetanensis*. Epidemiological investigations showed remarkable distributions of the protozoan infection in immunodeficient and diarrheic patients in Nigeria (Alakpa et al., 2002), Mexico (Jiménez-González et al., 2012), Honduras (Kaminsky et al., 2016), and Turkey (Karaman et al., 2015). The data summarized in Table 4.5 demonstrates that diarrhea is a major risk factor for *C. cayetanensis* infection in humans: both immunocompromised and immunocompetent individuals with diarrhea (7.38% vs 9.14%, respectively) had a significantly higher prevalence of infection than patients with other symptoms (4.91% vs 2.09%, respectively; $P = .0001$).

4.3.2 Age

Age may be another factor that affects the occurrence of cyclosporiasis in humans. Many studies have reported that children show a higher prevalence of *C. cayetanensis* infection than the general population in countries such as Guatemala, Nepal, Turkey, and Honduras, among others (Bern et al., 1999; Kimura et al., 2005; Erdogan et al., 2012; Bhandari et al., 2015; Kaminsky et al., 2016). However, unexpectedly, children had a lower infection rate than the general population (4.90% vs 9.36%, respectively) of immunocompetent

Table 4.5 Distributions of Cyclospora cayetanensis infection in different human population groups.

Population groups	Number of investigation samples	Number of positive	Prevalence [95 CI]
HIV/AIDS or immunodeficient with diarrhea	3863	285	7.38% [6.55–8.20]
Children	0	0	0
General	3863	285	7.38% [6.55–8.20]
HIV/AIDS or immunodeficient without diarrhea	5661	278	4.91% [4.35–5.47]
Children	364	17	4.67% [2.49–6.85]
General	5297	261	4.93% [4.34–5.51]
Individuals with diarrhea	26,852	2453	9.14% [8.79–9.48]
Children	1347	66	4.90% [3.75–6.05]
General	25,505	2387	9.36% [9.00–9.72]
Individuals without diarrhea	118,034	2462	2.09% [2.00–2.17]
Children	25,077	439	1.75% [1.59–1.91]
General	92,957	2023	2.18% [2.08–2.27]
Total	154,410	5478	3.55% [3.46–3.64]

Note: Summarized from "Table 4.3: Epidemiological investigation of *Cyclospora cayetanensis* infection in humans."

individuals with diarrhea, according to epidemiological statistics ($P < .0001$) (Table 4.5). This might be due to the fact that adult population consumes more raw produce than children, which is considered an important vehicle for *Cyclospora* oocysts transmission.

4.3.3 Hygiene and sanitary condition

Poor sanitation conditions are another risk factor for *C. cayetanensis* infection. The prevalence of infection is significantly higher in the people from low-income communities living in areas with poor sanitation, such as in Peru (54.88% and 41.58%), Venezuela (24.20%), and India (22.27%) (Burstein Alva, 2005; Nundy et al., 2011; Cazorla et al., 2012; Jeevitha et al., 2014). Similarly in Nepal, *Cyclospora* infection rates were higher in the members of a family that reared livestock at home than the families who did not (Bhandari et al., 2015).

4.3.4 Traveling

C. cayetanensis is also an important pathogen causing traveler's diarrhea, especially in industrialized regions (Mansfield and Gajadhar, 2004; Shields and Olson, 2003). International travel or expatriate relocation to developing countries with disease-endemic areas or poor sanitation might be a risk factor for cyclosporiasis in humans (Fryauff et al., 1999; Pandey et al., 2011; Kłudkowska et al., 2017).

4.3.5 Environmental factors

A pilot study sought to infect human volunteers with *C. cayetanensis*; however, no oocysts were detected in any stool samples during the 16-week trial in any of the seven volunteers (Alfano-Sobsey et al., 2004). Given the results of this study, the conditions necessary for *Cyclospora* to become infectious were likely not maintained when preparing or storing the oocysts. Further studies are necessary to assess effects of temperature, humidity, storage conditions, and disinfection on the survival, viability, and infectivity of stored *Cyclospora* oocysts.

4.4 Animal reservoirs

4.4.1 Nonhuman primates

Nonhuman primates (NHPs) harbor a number of *Cyclospora* species. *Cyclospora cercopitheci* in vervet monkeys (*Cercopithecus aethiops*), *C. colobi* in colobus monkeys (*Colobus guereza*), and *C. papionis* in olive baboons

(*Papio anubis*) were characterized in 1999 (Eberhard et al., 1999). Another species *C. macacae* was described in rhesus monkeys (*Macaca mulatta*) in 2015 (Li et al., 2015). Among the *Cyclospora* species reported in NHPs, the occurrence of *C. papionis* was 17.9% in the captured baboons in Kenya (Li et al., 2011) and occurrence of *C. macacae* was 6.8% in the rhesus monkeys in China (Li et al., 2015).

4.4.2 Other animals

Several *Cyclospora*-like organisms have been reported in various animals, including dogs, cattle, chickens, rats/house mice, birds, and shellfish (Table 4.6) (Eberhard et al., 2001; Ortega and Sanchez, 2010). The Asian freshwater clams (*Corbicula fluminea*) can recover oocysts of *C. cayetanensis* by artificial infection contamination, thus could be used as a biological indicator of water contamination with oocysts (Graczyk et al., 1998). In a study in Nepal, the households keeping livestock had higher *Cyclospora* infection rates (Bhandari et al., 2015), indicating the possible connection of the infection with domestic animals.

Another study attempted to develop an animal model for *C. cayetanensis* to study human cyclosporiasis. Various types of animal (various strains of mice, rats, sand rats, chickens, ducks, rabbits, birds, hamsters, ferrets, pigs, dogs, owl monkeys, rhesus monkeys, and cynomolgus monkeys) were inoculated with human-infecting *C. cayetanensis* oocysts by gavage. None of the animals developed patent infection or signs of infection 4–6 weeks after inoculation. It was concluded that none of the mammals tested are susceptible to infection with *C. cayetanensis* (Graczyk et al., 1998).

4.5 Search strategy and selection criteria

We searched PubMed, Web of Science, ScienceDirect, Wangfang, and the China National Knowledge Infrastructure, with no language restriction, using the following search terms to screen for relevant articles: "*Cyclospora*," "*Cyclospora*-like organisms," "cyclosporiasis," "cyanobacterium-like body," or "alga-like organism." For articles without the full text or published in other languages, the titles and abstracts in English were screened for mention of *Cyclospora* infection. We included articles published up to December 31, 2018, when calculating the epidemiological data and summarizing the cases of infection. Articles published in English, Spanish, Portuguese, French, Turkish, Chinese, Czech, Dutch, Japanese, Rumanian, and German were included (Fig. 4.2).

Table 4.6 *Cyclospora* spp. or *Cyclospora*-like organisms reported in various animals.

Countries (site)	Host	Sample number	Positive number	Prevalence	Detection method	References
Brazil, São Paulo	Dogs		2 cases		PCR–RFLP	Yai et al., 1997
China, Guangzhou	Dairy cattle		2 cases			Li et al., 2007
China	Dairy cattle	168	6	3.57%	PCR–OLA	Xiao et al., 2007
China, Shaanxi	Golden snub-nosed monkeys	71	2	2.82%	PCR	Zhao et al., 2013
China, Guangxi	Crab-eating macaques	205	1	0.49%	PCR	Ye et al., 2014
China, Guizhou	Rhesus monkeys	411	28	6.81%	PCR	Li et al., 2015
China	Monkeys	3349	7	0.21%	Light microscopy	Li et al., 2017b
Egypt	Dogs	130	1	0.77%	Light microscopy	Awadallah and Salem, 2015
Equatorial Guinea	Drills (*Mandrillus leucophaeus poensis*)	51	11	21.57%	PCR	Eberhard et al., 2014
Ethiopia	Baboons	59	8	13.56%	Modified Ziehl-Neelsen satin	Legesse and Erko, 2004
Ethiopia	Vervet monkeys	41	9	21.95%	Modified Ziehl-Neelsen satin	Legesse and Erko, 2004
India	Sheep	65	2	3.08%	Ziehl-Neelsen stain and confirmed with PCR	Basnett et al., 2018
India	Goat	216	4	1.85%	Ziehl-Neelsen stain and confirmed with PCR	Basnett et al., 2018
Italy	Monkeys	119	11	9.24%	qPCR	Marangi et al., 2015
Japan	Claves		3 cases		PCR	Yamada et al., 2014
Kenya	Nonhuman primates	511	81	15.85%	PCR	Eberhard et al., 2001
Kenya	Baboons	235	42	17.87%	PCR	Li et al., 2011

Location	Host	Number examined	Positive	Percentage	Method	Reference
Malaysia	Large-billed crow	106	6	5.66%	Modified Ziehl-Neelsen satin	Lee et al., 2008
Mexico	Chicken		1 case		Kinyoun's acid-fast stain; autofluorescence under UV	García-López et al., 1996
Nepal	Chicken	110	3	2.73%		Sherchand and Cross, 2001
Nepal	Dogs	90	2	2.22%		Sherchand and Cross, 2001
Nepal	Rats/House mice	50	2	4.00%		Sherchand and Cross, 2001
Nepal	Dog	14	2	14.29%	PCR	Chu et al., 2004
Nepal	Chicken	3	1	33.33%	PCR	Chu et al., 2004
Nepal	Monkey	3	1	33.33%	PCR	Chu et al., 2004
Spain	Birds	984	23	2.34%	Harada-Mori technique satin	Cordón et al., 2009
Spain	Nonhuman primates	18	6	33.33%	Modified Ziehl-Neelsen satin	Cordón et al., 2008
Spain	Carnivorous animals	72	3	4.17%	Modified Ziehl-Neelsen satin	Cordón et al., 2008
Spain	Artiodactyla animals	198	18	9.09%	Modified Ziehl-Neelsen satin	Cordón et al., 2008
Thailand, Samutprakarn	Cockroaches	920	10	1.09%	Modified acid-fast stain	Chamavit et al., 2011
Tanzania	Baboons		3 cases		PCR	Smith et al., 1996
Tunisia	Wild shellfish	1255	526	41.91%	qPCR	Ghozzi et al., 2017
Turkey (Bays of Izmir and Mersin)	Edible shellfish	53	14	26.42%	qPCR/HRM	Aksoy et al., 2014
US	Howler monkey	96	17	17.71%		Helenbrook et al., 2015
Total		**9603**	**847**	**8.82%**		

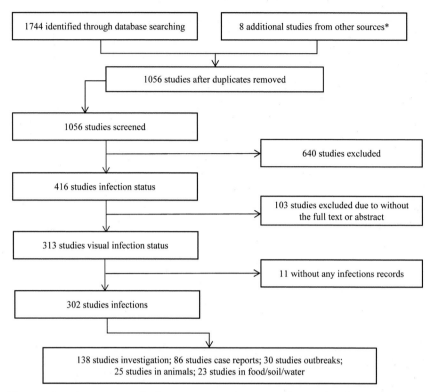

Fig. 4.2 Search strategy and selection criteria about prevalence of *Cyclospora*.

4.6 Conclusion

Human cyclosporiasis caused by *C. cayetanensis* was firstly reported in Papua New Guinea in 1979. Since then *C. cayetanensis* infections in humans have been reported in at least 54 countries of the world with a total number of 13,845 cases up to December 2018. Of the countries, more than 13 have recorded cyclosporiasis outbreaks with 6557 cases. The average prevalence of cyclosporiasis is 3.55% (5478/154,410) in humans worldwide. Detection of the pathogen is mostly based on oocyst morphology, staining, and molecular testing (PCR). *C. cayetanensis* infections are commonly reported in developing countries with low-socioeconomic levels or disease-endemic areas. However, large outbreaks commonly occurred in developed countries in Europe and the Americas, and among travelers from these countries and those returning from tropical endemic areas. Among susceptible populations, the highest prevalence has been documented in immunocompetent individuals with diarrhea. The marked seasonality of *C. cayetanensis* infection, which occurs predominantly during the rainy season or summer, is well documented. *Cyclospora* spp. or *Cyclospora*-like organisms are also reported in some animals.

References

Abanyie, F., Harvey, R.R., Harris, J.R., Wiegand, R.E., Gaul, L., Desvignes-Kendrick, M., Irvin, K., Williams, I., Hall, R.L., Herwaldt, B., Gray, E.B., Qvarnstrom, Y., Wise, M.E., Cantu, V., Cantey, P.T., Bosch, S., DA Silva, A.J., Fields, A., Bishop, H., Wellman, A., Beal, J., Wilson, N., Fiore, A.E., Tauxe, R., Lance, S., Slutsker, L., Parise, M., Multistate Cyclosporiasis Outbreak Investigation Team, 2015. 2013 multistate outbreaks of *Cyclospora cayetanensis* infections associated with fresh produce: focus on the Texas investigations. Epidemiol. Infect. 143, 3451–3458.

Abdel-Hafeez, E.H., Ahmad, A.K., Ali, B.A., Moslam, F.A., 2012. Opportunistic parasites among immunosuppressed children in Minia District, Egypt. Korean J. Parasitol. 50, 57–62.

Abou el Naga, I.F., 1999. Studies on a newly emerging protozoal pathogen: *Cyclospora cayetanensis*. J. Egypt. Soc. Parasitol. 29, 575–586.

Agholi, M., Hatam, G.R., Motazedian, M.H., 2013. HIV/AIDS-associated opportunistic protozoal diarrhea. AIDS Res. Hum. Retroviruses 29, 35–41.

Agholi, M., Shahabadi, S.N., Motazedian, M.H., Hatam, G.R., 2016. Prevalence of enteric protozoan oocysts with special reference to *Sarcocystis cruzi* among fecal samples of diarrheic immunodeficient patients in Iran. Korean J. Parasitol. 54, 339–344.

Ahmed, N.H., Chowdhary, A., 2013. Comparison of different methods of detection of enteric pathogenic protozoa. Indian J. Med. Microbiol. 31, 154–160.

Ahmed, N.H., Chowdhary, A., 2015. Pattern of co-infection by enteric pathogenic parasites among HIV sero-positive individuals in a tertiary care hospital, Mumbai, India. Indian J. Sex. Transm. Dis. AIDS 36, 40–47.

Aksoy, U., Akisu, C., Sahin, S., Usluca, S., Yalcin, G., Kuralay, F., Oral, A.M., 2007. First reported waterborne outbreak of *cryptosporidiosis* with *Cyclospora* co-infection in Turkey. Euro Surveill. 12, E070215.4.

Aksoy, U., Marangi, M., Papini, R., Ozkoc, S., Bayram Delibas, S., Giangaspero, A., 2014. Detection of toxoplasma gondii and *Cyclospora cayetanensis* in mytilus galloprovincialis from Izmir Province coast (Turkey) by real time PCR/high-resolution melting analysis (HRM). Food Microbiol. 44, 128–135.

Alakpa, G., Fagbenro-Beyioku, A.F., Clarke, S.C., 2002. *Cyclospora cayetanensis* in stools submitted to hospitals in Lagos, Nigeria. Int. J. Infect. Dis. 6, 314–318.

Alakpa, G.E., Clarke, S.C., Fagbenro-Beyioku, A.F., 2003. *Cyclospora cayetanensis* infection in Lagos, Nigeria. Clin. Microbiol. Infect. 9, 731–733.

Albert, M.J., Kabir, I., Azim, T., Hossain, A., Ansaruzzaman, M., Unicomb, L., 1994. Diarrhea associated with *Cyclospora* sp. in Bangladesh. Diagn. Microbiol. Infect. Dis. 19, 47–49.

Al-Braiken, F.A., Amin, A., Beeching, N.J., Hommel, M., Hart, C.A., 2003. Detection of *Cryptosporidium* amongst diarrhoeic and asymptomatic children in Jeddah, Saudi Arabia. Ann. Trop. Med. Parasitol. 97, 505–510.

Alemu, G., Alelign, D., Abossie, A., 2018. Prevalence of opportunistic intestinal parasites and associated factors among HIV patients while receiving ART at Arba Minch hospital in Southern Ethiopia: a cross-sectional study. Ethiop. J. Health Sci. 28, 147–156.

Alfano-Sobsey, E.M., Eberhard, M.L., Seed, J.R., Weber, D.J., Won, K.Y., Nace, E.K., Moe, C.L., 2004. Human challenge pilot study with *Cyclospora cayetanensis*. Emerg. Infect. Dis. 10, 726–728.

Ali, M.S., Mahmoud, L.A., Abaza, B.E., Ramadan, M.A., 2000. Intestinal spore-forming protozoa among patients suffering from chronic renal failure. J. Egypt. Soc. Parasitol. 30, 93–100.

Al-Megrin, W.A., 2010. Intestinal parasites infection among immunocompromised patients in Riyadh, Saudi Arabia. Pak. J. Biol. Sci. 13, 390–394.

Almeria, S., Cinar, H.N., Dubey, J.P., 2019. *Cyclospora cayetanensis* and cyclosporiasis: an update. Microorganisms 7, 317.

Amatya, R., Poudyal, N., Gurung, R., Khanal, B., 2011. Prevalence of cryptosporidium species in paediatric patients in eastern Nepal. Trop. Doct. 41, 36–37.

Arslan, M.O., Sari, B., Kulu, B., Mor, N., 2008. The prevalence of intestinal parasites in children brought to the Kars Maternal and Children's Hospital with complaints of gastrointestinal symptoms. Turkiye Parazitol. Derg. 32, 253–256 (Article in Turkish).

Ashford, R.W., 1979. Occurrence of an undescribed coccidian in man in Papua New Guinea. Ann. Trop. Med. Parasitol. 73, 497–500.

Asma, I., Johari, S., Sim, B.L., Lim, Y.A., 2011. How common is intestinal parasitism in HIV-infected patients in Malaysia? Trop. Biomed. 28, 400–410.

Awadallah, M.A., Salem, L.M., 2015. Zoonotic enteric parasites transmitted from dogs in Egypt with special concern to *Toxocara canis* infection. Vet. World 8, 946–957.

Ayala-Gaytán, J.J., Díaz-Olachea, C., Riojas-Montalvo, P., Palacios-Martínez, C., 2004. Cyclosporidiosis: clinical and diagnostic characteristics of an epidemic outbreak. Rev. Gastroenterol. Mex. 69, 226–229 (Article in Spanish).

Baiomy, A.M., Mohamed, K.A., Ghannam, M.A., Shahat, S.A., Al-Saadawy, A.S., 2010. Opportunistic parasitic infections among immunocompromised Egyptian patients. J. Egypt. Soc. Parasitol. 40, 797–808.

Basnett, K., Nagarajan, K., Soundararajan, C., Vairamuthu, S., Sudhakar Rao, G.V., 2018. Morphological and molecular identification of *Cyclospora* species in sheep and goat at Tamil Nadu, India. J. Parasit. Dis. 42, 604–607.

Bednarska, M., Bajer, A., Welc-Falęciak, R., Pawełas, A., 2015. *Cyclospora cayetanensis* infection in transplant traveller: a case report of outbreak. Parasit. Vectors 8, 411.

Bednarska, M., Jankowska, I., Pawelas, A., Bajer, A., Wolska-Kuśnierz, B., Wielopolska, M., Welc-Falęciak, R., 2018. Prevalence of *Cryptosporidium*, *Blastocystis*, and other opportunistic infections in patients with primary and acquired immunodeficiency. Parasitol. Res. 117, 2869–2879.

Behera, B., Mirdha, B.R., Makharia, G.K., Bhatnagar, S., Dattagupta, S., Samantaray, J.C., 2008. Parasites in patients with malabsorption syndrome: a clinical study in children and adults. Dig. Dis. Sci. 53, 672–679.

Bellagra, N., Ajana, F., Coignard, C., Caillaux, M., Mouton, Y., 1998. Co-infection with *Cryptosporidium* sp and *Cyclospora* sp in an AIDS stage HIV patient. Ann. Biol. Clin. 56, 476–478 (Article in French).

Berlin, O.G., Novak, S.M., Porschen, R.K., Long, E.G., Stelma, G.N., Schaeffer 3rd., F.W., 1994. Recovery of *Cyclospora* organisms from patients with prolonged diarrhea. Clin. Infect. Dis. 18, 606–609.

Bern, C., Hernandez, B., Lopez, M.B., Arrowood, M.J., de Mejia, M.A., de Merida, A.M., Hightower, A.W., Venczel, L., Herwaldt, B.L., Klein, R.E., 1999. Epidemiologic studies of *Cyclospora cayetanensis* in Guatemala. Emerg. Infect. Dis. 5, 766–774.

Bern, C., Hernandez, B., Lopez, M.B., Arrowood, M.J., De Merida, A.M., Klein, R.E., 2000. The contrasting epidemiology of *Cyclospora* and *Cryptosporidium* among outpatients in Guatemala. Am. J. Trop. Med. Hyg. 63, 231–235.

Bern, C., Ortega, Y., Checkley, W., Roberts, J.M., Lescano, A.G., Cabrera, L., Verastegui, M., Black, R.E., Sterling, C., Gilman, R.H., 2002. Epidemiologic differences between cyclosporiasis and cryptosporidiosis in Peruvian children. Emerg. Infect. Dis. 8, 581–585.

Bhandari, D., Tandukar, S., Parajuli, H., Thapa, P., Chaudhary, P., Shrestha, D., Shah, P.K., Sherchan, J.B., Sherchand, J.B., 2015. *Cyclospora* infection among school children in Kathmandu, Nepal: prevalence and associated risk factors. Trop. Med. Health. 43, 211–216.

Bhattachan, B., Sherchand, J.B., Tandukar, S., Dhoubhadel, B.G., Gauchan, L., Rai, G., 2017. Detection of *Cryptosporidium parvum* and *Cyclospora cayetanensis* infections among people living in a slum area in Kathmandu valley, Nepal. BMC. Res. Notes 10, 464.

Birdal Akış, F., Beyhan, Y.E., 2018. Distribution of intestinal parasites in patients hospitalized in child intensive care unit. Turkiye Parazitol. Derg. 42, 113–117.

Blans, M.C., Ridwan, B.U., Verweij, J.J., Rozenberg-Arska, M., Verhoef, J., 2005. Cyclosporiasis outbreak, Indonesia. Emerg. Infect. Dis. 11, 1453–1455.

Borges, J.D., Alarcón, R.S., Neto, V.A., Gakiya, E., 2009. Intestinal parasitosis in Indians of the Mapuera community (Oriximiná, State of Pará, Brazil): high prevalence of *Blastocystis hominis* and finding of *Cryptosporidium* sp and *Cyclospora cayetanensis*. Rev. Soc. Bras. Med. Trop. 42, 348–350 (Article in Portuguese).

Botero-Garcés, J., Montoya-Palacio, M.N., Barguil, J.I., Castaño-González, A., 2006. An outbreak of *Cyclospora cayetanensis* in Medellín, Colombia. Rev. Salud Publica. (Bogota) 8, 258–268 (Article in Spanish).

Bourée, P., Lancon, A., Bisaro, F., Bonnot, G., 2007. Six human cyclosporiasis: with general review. J. Egypt. Soc. Parasitol. 37, 349–360.

Burrell, C., Reddy, S., Haywood, G., Cunningham, R., 2007. Cardiac arrest associated with febrile illness due to U.K. acquired *Cyclospora* cayetanensis. J. Inf. Secur. 54, e13–e15.

Burstein Alva, S., 2005. Cyclosporosis: an emergent parasitosis. (I) Clinical and epidemiological aspects. Rev. Gastroenterol. Peru 25, 328–335 (Article in Spanish).

Butcher, A.R., Lumb, R., Coulter, E., Nielsen, D.J., 1994. Coccidian/cyanobacterium-like body associated diarrhea in an Australian traveller returning from overseas. Pathology 26, 59–61.

Caramello, P., Brancale, T., Forno, B., Lucchini, A., Macor, A., Mazzucco, G., Tettoni, C., Ullio, A., 1995. Clinical and diagnostic aspects of travelers' diarrhea due to *Cyclospora* organisms. J. Travel Med. 2, 232–234.

Casillas, S.M., Bennett, C., Straily, A., 2018. Notes from the field: multiple cyclosporiasis outbreaks—United States, 2018. MMWR Morb. Mortal. Wkly Rep. 67, 1101–1102.

Cazorla, D., Acosta, M.E., Acosta, M.E., Morales, P., 2012. Clinical and epidemiological study of intestinal coccidioses in a rural population of a semiarid region from Falcon state, Venezuela. Invest. Clin. 53, 273–288 (Article in Spanish).

Cegielski, J.P., Ortega, Y.R., McKee, S., Madden, J.F., Gaido, L., Schwartz, D.A., Manji, K., Jorgensen, A.F., Miller, S.E., Pulipaka, U.P., Msengi, A.E., Mwakyusa, D.H., Sterling, C.R., Reller, L.B., 1999. *Cryptosporidium, enterocytozoon,* and *cyclospora* infections in pediatric and adult patients with diarrhea in Tanzania. Clin. Infect. Dis. 28, 314–321.

Centers for Disease Control and Prevention (CDC), 1997a. Outbreaks of cyclosporiasis—United States, 1997. MMWR Morb. Mortal. Wkly Rep. 46, 451–452.

Centers for Disease Control and Prevention (CDC), 1997b. Outbreak of cyclosporiasis—northern Virginia-Washington, D.C.-Baltimore, Maryland, metropolitan area, 1997. MMWR Morb. Mortal. Wkly Rep. 46, 689–691.

Centers for Disease Control and Prevention (CDC), 1998. Outbreak of cyclosporiasis—Ontario, Canada, May 1998. MMWR Morb. Mortal. Wkly Rep. 47, 806–809.

Centers for Disease Control and Prevention (CDC), 2004. Outbreak of cyclosporiasis associated with snow peas—Pennsylvania, 2004. MMWR Morb. Mortal. Wkly Rep. 53, 876–878.

Centers for Disease Control and Prevention (CDC), 2013. Outbreaks of cyclosporiasis—United States, June-August 2013. MMWR Morb. Mortal. Wkly Rep. 62, 862.

Chacín-Bonilla, L., Estévez, J., Monsalve, F., Quijada, L., 2001. *Cyclospora cayetanensis* infections among diarrheal patients from Venezuela. Am. J. Trop. Med. Hyg. 65, 351–354.

Chacín-Bonilla, L., Mejia de Young, M., Estevez, J., 2003. Prevalence and pathogenic role of *Cyclospora cayetanensis* in a Venezuelan community. Am. J. Trop. Med. Hyg. 68, 304–306.

Chacín-Bonilla, L., Barrios, F., Sanchez, Y., 2007. Epidemiology of *Cyclospora cayetanensis* infection in San Carlos Island, Venezuela: strong association between socio-economic status and infection. Trans. R. Soc. Trop. Med. Hyg. 101, 1018–1024.

Chakrabarti, P., Samantaray, J.C., Malik, S., 2004. Mixed infection with three intestinal coccidian parasites in an AIDS patient. J. Assoc. Physicians India 52, 975.

Chamavit, P., Sahaisook, P., Niamnuy, N., 2011. The majority of cockroaches from the Samutprakarn province of Thailand are carriers of parasitic organisms. EXCLI J. 10, 218–222.

Chokephaibulkit, K., Wanachiwanawin, D., Tosasuk, K., Vanprapa, N., Chearskul, S., 2001. A report case of *Cyclospora* and *Cryptosporidium* mixed infection in a HIV-negative child in Thailand. J. Med. Assoc. Thai. 84, 589–592.

Chopra, R.D., Dworkin, M.S., 2013. Descriptive epidemiology of enteric disease in Chennai, India. Epidemiol. Infect. 141, 953–957.

Chu, D.M., Sherchand, J.B., Cross, J.H., Orlandi, P.A., 2004. Detection of *Cyclospora cayetanensis* in animal fecal isolates from Nepal using an FTA filter-base polymerase chain reaction method. Am. J. Trop. Med. Hyg. 71, 373–379.

Ciçek, M., Uçmak, F., Ozekinci, T., 2011. Two diarrhea cases caused by *Cyclospora cayetanensis*. Mikrobiyol. Bul. 45, 553–557 (Article in Turkish).

Clarke, S.C., McIntyre, M., 1996. The incidence of *Cyclospora cayetanensis* in stool samples submitted to a district general hospital. Epidemiol. Infect. 117, 189–193.

Cordón, G.P., Prados, A.H., Romero, D., Moreno, M.S., Pontes, A., Osuna, A., Rosales, M.J., 2008. Intestinal parasitism in the animals of the zoological garden "Peña Escrita" (Almuñecar, Spain). Vet. Parasitol. 156, 302–309.

Cordón, G.P., Prados, A.H., Romero, D., Moreno, M.S., Pontes, A., Osuna, A., Rosales, M.J., 2009. Intestinal and haematic parasitism in the birds of the Almuñecar (Granada, Spain) ornithological garden. Vet. Parasitol. 165, 361–366.

Cordova Paz Soldan, O., Vargas Vásquez, F., Gonzalez Varas, A., Peréz Cordón, G., Velasco Soto, J.R., Sánchez-Moreno, M., Rodríguez Gonzalez, I., Rosales Lombardo, M.J., 2006. Intestinal parasitism in Peruvian children and molecular characterization of *Cryptosporidium* species. Parasitol. Res. 98, 576–581.

Crowley, B., Path, C., Moloney, C., Keane, C.T., 1996. *Cyclospora* species—a cause of diarrhoea among Irish travellers to Asia. Ir. Med. J. 89, 110–112.

de Górgolas, M., Fortés, J., Fernández Guerrero, M.L., 2001. *Cyclospora cayetanensis* Cholecystitis in a patient with AIDS. Ann. Intern. Med. 134, 166.

de Paz, V.C., Brínguez, M.B., Viamonte, B.V., Suárez, C.L., Rodríguez, A.M., Martiñex, Z.A., 2003. Diagnosis of coccidia and microspores in specimens of diarrheal feces from Cuban HIV seropositive patients: first report of microspores in Cuba. Rev. Cubana Med. Trop. 55, 14–18 (Article in Spanish).

Değirmenci, A., Sevil, N., Güneş, K., Yolasiğmaz, A., Turgay, N., 2007. Distribution of intestinal parasites detected in the parasitology laboratory of the Ege University Medical School Hospital, in 2005. Turkiye Parazitol. Derg. 31, 133–135 (Article in Turkish).

Dekker, E., Kager, P.A., 2002. Prolonged diarrhea and weight loss after a biking trip from Tibet to Nepal: infection with *Cyclospora*. Ned. Tijdschr. Geneeskd. 146, 1502–1504 (Article in Dutch).

Deluol, A.M., Junod, C.H., 1996. *Cyclospora* sp. Ann. Biol. Clin. 54, 373–379 (Article in French).

Deodhar, L., Maniar, J.K., Saple, D.G., 2000. *Cyclospora* infection in acquired immunodeficiency syndrome. J. Assoc. Physicians India 48, 404–406.

Devera, R., Blanco,Y., Cabello, E., 2005. High prevalence of *Cyclospora cayetanensis* among indigenous people in Bolivar State,Venezuela. Cad. Saude Publica 21, 1778–1784 (Article in Spanish).

Di Gliullo, A.B., Cribari, M.S., Bava, A.J., Cicconetti, J.S., Collazos, R., 2000. *Cyclospora cayetanensis* in sputum and stool samples. Rev. Inst. Med.Trop. Sao Paulo 42, 115–117.

Diaz, E., Mondragon, J., Ramirez, E., Bernal, R., 2003. Epidemiology and control of intestinal parasites with nitazoxanide in children in Mexico. Am. J. Trop. Med. Hyg. 68, 384–385.

Dillingham, R.A., Pinkerton, R., Leger, P., Severe, P., Guerrant, R.L., Pape, J.W., Fitzgerald, D.W., 2009. High early mortality in patients with chronic acquired immunodeficiency syndrome diarrhea initiating antiretroviral therapy in Haiti: a case-control study. Am. J. Trop. Med. Hyg. 80, 1060–1064.

Doğan, N., Oz,Y., Koçman, N.U., Nursal, A.F., 2012. Comparison of individual differences in the direct microscopic examination in the diagnosis of intestinal parasites. Turkiye Parazitol. Derg. 36, 211–214 (Article in Turkish).

Döller, P.C., Dietrich, K., Filipp, N., Brockmann, S., Dreweck, C., Vonthein, R., Wagner-Wiening, C., Wiedenmann, A., 2002. Cyclosporiasis outbreak in Germany associated with the consumption of salad. Emerg. Infect. Dis. 8, 992–994.

Drenaggi, D., Cirioni, O., Giacometti, A., Fiorentini, A., Scalise, G., 1998. Cyclosporiasis in a traveler returning from South America. J.Travel Med. 5, 153–155.

Easow, J.M., Mukhopadhyay, C., Wilson, G., Guha, S., Jalan, B.Y., Shivananda, P.G., 2005. Emerging opportunistic protozoa and intestinal pathogenic protozoal infestation profile in children of western Nepal. Nepal Med. Coll. J. 7, 134–137.

Eassa, S.M., El-Wahab, E.W., Lotfi, S.E., El Masry, S.A., Shatat, H.Z., Kotkat, A.M., 2016. Risk factors associated with parasitic infection among municipality solid-waste workers in an Egyptian community. J. Parasitol. 102, 214–221.

Eberhard, M.L., Nace, E.K., Freeman, A.R., Streit, T.G., da Silva, A.J., Lammie, P.J., 1999. *Cyclospora cayetanensis* infections in Haiti: a common occurrence in the absence of watery diarrhea. Am. J.Trop. Med. Hyg. 60, 584–586.

Eberhard, M.L., Njenga, M.N., DaSilva, A.J., Owino, D., Nace, E.K., Won, K.Y., Mwenda, J.M., 2001. A survey for *Cyclospora* spp. in Kenyan primates, with some notes on its biology. J. Parasitol. 87, 1394–1397.

Eberhard, M.L., Owens, J.R., Bishop, H.S., de Almeida, M.E., da Silva, A.J., 2014. *Cyclospora* spp. in drills, Bioko Island, Equatorial Guinea. Emerg. Infect. Dis. 20, 510–511.

Egloff, N., Oehler, T., Rossi, M., Nguyen, X.M., Furrer, H., 2001. Chronic watery diarrhea due to co-infection with *Cryptosporidium* spp and *Cyclospora cayetanensis* in a Swiss AIDS patient traveling in Thailand. J.Travel Med. 8, 143–145.

El Fatni, C., Olmo, F., El Fatni, H., Romero, D., Rosales, M.J., 2014. First genotyping of *Giardia duodenalis* and prevalence of enteroparasites in children from Tetouan (Morocco). Parasite 21, 48.

El Naga, I.F., Negm, A.Y., Awadalla, H.N., 1998. Preliminary identification of an intestinal coccidian parasite in man. J. Egypt. Soc. Parasitol. 28, 807–814.

El Naggar, H.H., Handousa, A.E., El Hamshary, E.M., El Shazly, A.M., 1999. Evaluation of five stains in diagnosing human intestinal coccidiosis. J. Egypt. Soc. Parasitol. 29, 883–891.

El Shazly, A.M., Awad, S.E., Sultan, D.M., Sadek, G.S., Khalil, H.H., Morsy, T.A., 2006. Intestinal parasites in Dakahlia governorate, with different techniques in diagnosing protozoa. J. Egypt. Soc. Parasitol. 36, 1023–1034.

Erdogan, D.D., Kurt, O., Mandıracıoglu, A., Uner, A., Ak, M., Dagci, H., 2012. Prevalence and associated factors of *Cryptosporidium* spp. and *Cyclospora cayetanensis* in Izmir province, Turkey. Kafkas Üniversitesi Veteriner Fakültesi Dergisi 18, A105–A110.

Escobedo, A.A., Núñez, F.A., 1999. Prevalence of intestinal parasites in Cuban acquired immunodeficiency syndrome (AIDS) patients. Acta Trop. 72, 125–130.

Estran, C., Chaillou, S., Marty, P., 2004. Parasitism risk for tourists in the Dominican Republic: *Cyclospora*. Med. Trop. 64, 98–99 (Article in French).

Fernandes, A.O., Carollo, M.C., Braz, L.M., Amato Neto, V., Villela, M.S., 1998. Human cyclosporiasis diagnosis: report of a case in São Paulo, SP, Brazil. Rev. Inst. Med. Trop. Sao Paulo 40, 391–394.

Fregonesi, B.M., Suzuki, M.N., Machado, C.S., Tonani, K.A., Fernandes, A.P., Monroe, A.A., Cervi, M.C., Segura-Muñoz, S., 2015. Emergent and re-emergent parasites in HIV-infected children: immunological and socio-environmental conditions that are involved in the transmission of *Giardia* spp. and *Cryptosporidium* spp. Rev. Soc. Bras. Med. Trop. 48, 753–758.

Frickmann, H., Schwarz, N.G., Rakotozandrindrainy, R., May, J., Hagen, R.M., 2015. PCR for enteric pathogens in high-prevalence settings. What does a positive signal tell us? Infect. Dis. 47, 491–498.

Fryauff, D.J., Krippner, R., Prodjodipuro, P., Ewald, C., Kawengian, S., Pegelow, K., Yun, T., von Heydwolff-Wehnert, C., Oyofo, B., Gross, R., 1999. *Cyclospora cayetanensis* among expatriate and indigenous populations of West Java, Indonesia. Emerg. Infect. Dis. 5, 585–588.

García-López, H.L., Rodríguez-Tovar, L.E., Medina-De la Garza, C.E., 1996. Identification of *Cyclospora* in poultry. Emerg. Infect. Dis. 2, 356–357.

Gascón, J., Corachan, M., Bombi, J.A., Valls, M.E., Bordes, J.M., 1995. *Cyclospora* in patients with traveller's diarrhea. Scand. J. Infect. Dis. 27, 511–514.

Gascón, J., Alvarez, M., Eugènia Valls, M., Maria Bordas, J., Teresa Jiménez De Anta, M., Corachán, M., 2001. Cyclosporiasis: a clinical and epidemiological study in travellers with imported *Cyclospora cayetanensis* infection. Med. Clin. (Barc.) 116, 461–464 (Article in Spanish).

Ghozzi, K., Marangi, M., Papini, R., Lahmar, I., Challouf, R., Houas, N., Ben Dhiab, R., Normanno, G., Babba, H., Giangaspero, A., 2017. First report of Tunisian coastal water contamination by protozoan parasites using mollusk bivalves as biological indicators. Mar. Pollut. Bull. 117, 197–202.

Giangaspero, A., Gasser, R.B., 2019. Human cyclosporiasis. Lancet Infect. Dis. 19, e226–e236.

Giangaspero, A., Marangi, M., Koehler, A.V., Papini, R., Normanno, G., Lacasella, V., Lonigro, A., Gasser, R.B., 2015. Molecular detection of *Cyclospora* in water, soil, vegetables and humans in southern Italy signals a need for improved monitoring by health authorities. Int. J. Food Microbiol. 211, 95–100.

Gibbs, R.A., Nanyonjo, R., Pingault, N.M., Combs, B.G., Mazzucchelli, T., Armstrong, P., Tarling, G., Dowse, G.K., 2013. An outbreak of *Cyclospora* infection on a cruise ship. Epidemiol. Infect. 141, 508–516.

Gonçalves, E.M., Uemura, I.H., Castilho, V.L., Corbett, C.E., 2005. Retrospective study of the occurrence of *Cyclospora cayetanensis* at Clinical Hospital of the University of São Paulo Medical School, SP. Rev. Soc. Bras. Med. Trop. 38, 326–330.

Graczyk, T.K., Ortega, Y.R., Conn, D.B., 1998. Recovery of waterborne oocysts of *Cyclospora cayetanensis* by Asian freshwater clams (*Corbicula fluminea*). Am. J. Trop. Med. Hyg. 59, 928–932.

Green, S.T., McKendrick, M.W., Mohsen, A.H., Schmid, M.L., Prakasam, S.F., 2000. Two simultaneous cases of *Cyclospora* cayatensis enteritis returning from the Dominican Republic. J. Travel Med. 7, 41–42.

Gupta, A.K., 2011. Intestinal coccidian parasitic infections in rural community in and around Loni, Maharashtra. J. Parasit. Dis. 35, 54–56.

Gupta, S., Narang, S., Nunavath, V., Singh, S., 2008. Chronic diarrhoea in HIV patients: prevalence of coccidian parasites. Indian J. Med. Microbiol. 26, 172–175.

Hall, R.L., Jones, J.L., Herwaldt, B.L., 2011. Surveillance for laboratory-confirmed sporadic cases of cyclosporiasis—United States, 1997–2008. MMWR Surveill. Summ. 60, 1–11.

Hawash,Y.A., Dorgham, L.S., Amir, e.-A.M., Sharaf, O.F., 2015. Prevalence of intestinal protozoa among Saudi patients with chronic renal failure: a case-control study. J. Trop. Med. 2015, 563478.

Helenbrook, W.D., Wade, S.E., Shields, W.M., Stehman, S.V., Whipps, C.M., 2015. Gastrointestinal parasites of ecuadorian mantled howler monkeys (*Alouatta palliata aequatorialis*) based on fecal analysis. J. Parasitol. 101, 341–350.

Helmy, M.M., Rashed, L.A., Abdel-Fattah, H.S., 2006. Co-infection with *Cryptosporidium parvum* and *Cyclospora cayetanensis* in immunocompromised patients. J. Egypt. Soc. Parasitol. 36, 613–627.

Herwaldt, B.L., 2000. *Cyclospora cayetanensis*: a review, focusing on the outbreaks of cyclosporiasis in the 1990s. Clin. Infect. Dis. 31, 1040–1057.

Herwaldt, B.L., Ackers, M.L., 1997. An outbreak in 1996 of cyclosporiasis associated with imported raspberries. The Cyclospora Working Group. N. Engl. J. Med. 336, 1548–1556.

Herwaldt, B.L., Beach, M.J., 1999. The return of *Cyclospora* in 1997: another outbreak of cyclosporiasis in North America associated with imported raspberries. Cyclospora Working Group. Ann. Intern. Med. 130, 210–220.

Ho, A.Y., Lopez, A.S., Eberhart, M.G., Levenson, R., Finkel, B.S., da Silva, A.J., Roberts, J.M., Orlandi, P.A., Johnson, C.C., Herwaldt, B.L., 2002. Outbreak of cyclosporiasis associated with imported raspberries, Philadelphia, Pennsylvania, 2000. Emerg. Infect. Dis. 8, 783–788.

Hoang, L.M., Fyfe, M., Ong, C., Harb, J., Champagne, S., Dixon, B., Isaac-Renton, J., 2005. Outbreak of cyclosporiasis in British Columbia associated with imported Thai basil. Epidemiol. Infect. 133, 23–27.

Hoge, C.W., Echeverria, P., Rajah, R., Jacobs, J., Malthouse, S., Chapman, E., Jimenez, L.M., Shlim, D.R., 1995. Prevalence of *Cyclospora* species and other enteric pathogens among children less than 5 years of age in Nepal. J. Clin. Microbiol. 33, 3058–3060.

Huang, P., Weber, J.T., Sosin, D.M., Griffin, P.M., Long, E.G., Murphy, J.J., Kocka, F., Peters, C., Kallick, C., 1995. The first reported outbreak of diarrheal illness associated with *Cyclospora* in the United States. Ann. Intern. Med. 123, 409–414.

Hussein, E.M., 2007. Molecular identification of *Cycospora* spp. using multiplex PCR from diarrheic children compared to others conventional methods. J. Egypt. Soc. Parasitol. 37, 585–598.

Hussein, E.M., Abdul-Manaem, A.H., el-Attary, S.L., 2005. *Cyclospora* cayetanensis oocysts in sputum of a patient with active pulmonary tuberculosis, case report in Ismailia, Egypt. J. Egypt. Soc. Parasitol. 35, 787–793.

Hussein, E.M., El-Moamly, A.A., Dawoud, H.A., Fahmy, H., El-Shal, H.E., Sabek, N.A., 2007. Real-time PCR and flow cytometry in detection of *Cyclospora* oocysts in fecal samples of symptomatic and asymptomatic pediatrics patients. J. Egypt. Soc. Parasitol. 37, 151–170.

Insulander, M., Svenungsson, B., Lebbad, M., Karlsson, L., de Jong, B., 2010. A foodborne outbreak of *Cyclospora* infection in Stockholm, Sweden. Foodborne Pathog. Dis. 7, 1585–1587.

Iqbal, J., Hira, P.R., Al-Ali, F., Khalid, N., 2011. *Cyclospora cayetanensis*: first report of imported and autochthonous infections in Kuwait. J. Infect. Dev. Ctries. 5, 383–390.

Iyer, R.N., 2006. Cyclosporiasis in an infant. Indian J. Med. Microbiol. 24, 144–145.

Jayshree, R.S., Acharya, R.S., Sridhar, H., 1998. *Cyclospora cayetanensis*-associated diarrhoea in a patient with acute myeloid leukaemia. J. Diarrhoeal Dis. Res. 16, 254–255.

Jeevitha, D., Pushparaj, S.P., Kanchana, M., 2014. Comparative study of the prevalence of intestinal parasites in low socioeconomic areas from South Chennai, India. J. Parasitol. Res. 2014, 630968.

Jelinek, T., Lotze, M., Eichenlaub, S., Löscher, T., Nothdurft, H.D., 1997. Prevalence of infection with *Cryptosporidium parvum* and *Cyclospora cayetanensis* among international travellers. Gut 41, 801–804.

Jelínková, A., Kašičková, D., Valkoun, A., 2011. *Cyclospora cayetanensis*—the rare causal agent of diarrhoeal diseases. Klin. Mikrobiol. Infekc. Lek. 17, 86–88 (Article in Czech).

Jiang, Y., Yuan, Z., Zang, G., Li, D., Wang, Y., Zhang, Y., Liu, H., Cao, J., Shen, Y., 2018. *Cyclospora cayetanensis* infections among diarrheal outpatients in Shanghai: a retrospective case study. Front. Med. 12, 98–103.

Jiménez-González, G.B., Martínez-Gordillo, M.N., Caballero-Salazar, S., Peralta-Abarca, G.E., Cárdenas-Cardoz, R., Arzate-Barbosa, P., Ponce-Macotela, M., 2012. Microsporidia in pediatric patients with leukemia or limphoma. Rev. Invest. Clin. 64, 25–31 (Article in Spanish).

Junod, C., Deluol, A.M., Cosnes, J., Bauer, P., 1994. *Cyclospora*, a new coccidium agent of travelers' diarrhea. 11 cases. Presse Med. 23, 1312 (Article in French).

Kaminsky, R.G., Lagos, J., Raudales Santos, G., Urrutia, S., 2016. Marked seasonality of *Cyclospora cayetanensis* infections: ten-year observation of hospital cases, Honduras. BMC Infect. Dis. 16, 66.

Kansouzidou, A., Charitidou, C., Varnis, T., Vavatsi, N., Kamaria, F., 2004. *Cyclospora cayetanensis* in a patient with travelers' diarrhea: case report and review. J. Travel Med. 11, 61–63.

Karaman, U., Daldal, N., Ozer, A., Enginyurt, O., Erturk, O., 2015. Epidemiology of *Cyclospora* species in humans in Malatya Province in Turkey. Jundishapur J. Microbiol. 8, e18661.

Kasper, M.R., Lescano, A.G., Lucas, C., Gilles, D., Biese, B.J., Stolovitz, G., Reaves, E.J., 2012. Diarrhea outbreak during U.S. military training in El Salvador. PLoS ONE 7, e40404.

Khanaliha, K., Mohebali, M., Davoudi, S., Reza Hosseini, O., Tarighi, F., Rezaeian, T., Rezaeian, M., 2015. Detection of emergence *Cyclospora cayetanensis* in A HIV(+)/AIDS patient with diarrhea from Tehran: a case report. Iran J. Public Health 44, 865–868.

Kimura, K., Rai, S.K., Rai, G., Insisiengmay, S., Kawabata, M., Karanis, P., Uga, S., 2005. Study on *Cyclospora cayetanensis* associated with diarrheal disease in Nepal and Loa PDR. Southeast Asian J. Trop. Med. Public Health 36, 1371–1376.

Kitajima, M., Haramoto, E., Iker, B.C., Gerba, C.P., 2014. Occurrence of *Cryptosporidium*, *Giardia*, and *Cyclospora* in influent and effluent water at wastewater treatment plants in Arizona. Sci. Total Environ. 484, 129–136.

Kłudkowska, M., Pielok, Ł., Frąckowiak, K., Paul, M., 2017. Intestinal coccidian parasites as an underestimated cause of travellers' diarrhoea in Polish immunocompetent patients. Acta Parasitol. 62, 630–638.

Koru, O., Araz, E., Inci, A., Tanyuksel, M., 2006. Co-infection of *Giardia* intestinalis and *Cyclospora* cayetanensis in an immunocompetent patient with prolonged diarrhea: case report. J. Microbiol. 44, 360–362.

Kozak, G.K., MacDonald, D., Landry, L., Farber, J.M., 2013. Foodborne outbreaks in Canada linked to produce: 2001 through 2009. J. Food Prot. 76, 173–183.

Kulkarni, S.V., Kairon, R., Sane, S.S., Padmawar, P.S., Kale, V.A., Thakar, M.R., Mehendale, S.M., Risbud, A.R., 2009. Opportunistic parasitic infections in HIV/AIDS patients presenting with diarrhoea by the level of immunesuppression. Indian J. Med. Res. 130, 63–66.

Kumar, S.S., Ananthan, S., Lakshmi, P., 2002a. Intestinal parasitic infection in HIV infected patients with diarrhoea in Chennai. Indian J. Med. Microbiol. 20, 88–91.

Kumar, S.S., Ananthan, S., Saravanan, P., 2002b. Role of coccidian parasites in causation of diarrhoea in HIV infected patients in Chennai. Indian J. Med. Res. 116, 85–89.

Kumar, P., Vats, O., Kumar, D., Singh, S., 2017. Coccidian intestinal parasites among immunocompetent children presenting with diarrhea: are we missing them? Trop. Parasitol. 7, 37–40.

Kurniawan, A., Karyadi, T., Dwintasari, S.W., Sari, I.P., Yunihastuti, E., Djauzi, S., Smith, H.V., 2009. Intestinal parasitic infections in HIV/AIDS patients presenting with diarrhoea in Jakarta, Indonesia. Trans. R. Soc. Trop. Med. Hyg. 103, 892–898.

Lalonde, L.F., Reyes, J., Gajadhar, A.A., 2013. Application of a qPCR assay with melting curve analysis for detection and differentiation of protozoan oocysts in human fecal samples from Dominican Republic. Am. J. Trop. Med. Hyg. 89, 892–898.

Lammers, H.A., van Gool, T., Eeftinck Schattenkerk, J.K., 1996. 2 patients with diarrhea caused by *Cyclospora cayetanensis* following a trip to the tropics. Ned.Tijdschr. Geneeskd. 140, 890–892 (Article in Dutch).

Lee, H.Y., Stephen, A., Sushela, D., Mala, M., 2008. Detection of protozoan and bacterial pathogens of public health importance in faeces of *Corvus* spp. (large-billed crow). Trop. Biomed. 25, 134–139.

Legesse, M., Erko, B., 2004. Zoonotic intestinal parasites in *Papio anubis* (baboon) and *Cercopithecus aethiops* (vervet) from four localities in Ethiopia. Acta Trop. 90, 231–236.

Li, G., Xiao, S., Zhou, R., Li, W., Wadeh, H., 2007. Molecular characterization of *Cyclospora*-like organism from dairy cattle. Parasitol. Res. 100, 955–961.

Li, W., Kiulia, N.M., Mwenda, J.M., Nyachieo, A., Taylor, M.B., Zhang, X., Xiao, L., 2011. *Cyclospora papionis*, *Cryptosporidium hominis*, and human-pathogenic *Enterocytozoon bieneusi* in captive baboons in Kenya. J. Clin. Microbiol. 49, 4326–4329.

Li, N., Ye, J., Arrowood, M.J., Ma, J., Wang, L., Xu, H., Feng, Y., Xiao, L., 2015. Identification and morphologic and molecular characterization of *Cyclospora macacae* n. sp. from rhesus monkeys in China. Parasitol. Res. 114, 1811–1816.

Li, J., Chang, Y., Shi, K., Wang, R., Fu, K., Li, S., Xu, J., Jia, L., Guo, Z., Zhang, L., 2017a. Multilocus sequence typing and clonal population genetic structure of *Cyclospora cayetanensis* in humans. Parasitology 144, 1890–1897.

Li, J., Dong, H., Wang, R., Yu, F., Wu, Y., Chang, Y., Wang, C., Qi, M., Zhang, L., 2017b. An investigation of parasitic infections and review of molecular characterization of the intestinal protozoa in nonhuman primates in China from 2009 to 2015. Int. J. Parasitol. Parasites Wildl. 6, 8–15.

Li, J., Wang, R., Chen, Y., Xiao, L., Zhang, L., 2020. *Cyclospora cayetanensis* infection in humans: biological characteristics, clinical features, epidemiology, detection method, and treatment. Parasitology 147, 160–170.

Llanes, R., Velázquez, B., Reyes, Z., Somarriba, L., 2013. Co-infection with *Cyclospora cayetanensis* and *Salmonella typhi* in a patient with HIV infection and chronic diarrhoea. Pathog. Glob. Health. 107, 38–39.

Lopez, A.S., Dodson, D.R., Arrowood, M.J., Orlandi Jr., P.A., da Silva, A.J., Bier, J.W., Hanauer, S.D., Kuster, R.L., Oltman, S., Baldwin, M.S., Won, K.Y., Nace, E.M., Eberhard, M.L., Herwaldt, B.L., 2001. Outbreak of cyclosporiasis associated with basil in Missouri in 1999. Clin. Infect. Dis. 32, 1010–1017.

Lopez, A.S., Bendik, J.M., Alliance, J.Y., Roberts, J.M., da Silva, A.J., Moura, I.N., Arrowood, M.J., Eberhard, M.L., Herwaldt, B.L., 2003. Epidemiology of *Cyclospora cayetanensis* and other intestinal parasites in a community in Haiti. J. Clin. Microbiol. 41, 2047–2054.

Madico, G., McDonald, J., Gilman, R.H., Cabrera, L., Sterling, C.R., 1997. Epidemiology and treatment of *Cyclospora cayetanensis* infection in Peruvian children. Clin. Infect. Dis. 24, 977–981.

Madrid, V., Torrejón, E., Rivera, N., Madrid, M., 1998. *Cyclosporosis*. Report of a clinical case in Concepción, Chile. Rev. Med. Chil. 126, 559–562 (Article in Spanish).

Maggi, P., Brandonisio, O., Larocca, A.M., Rollo, M., Panaro, M.A., Marangi, A., Marzo, R., Angarano, G., Pastore, G., 1995. *Cyclospora* in AIDS patients: not always an agent of diarrhoic syndrome. New Microbiol. 18, 73–76.

Manatsathit, S., Tansupasawasdikul, S., Wanachiwanawin, D., Setawarin, S., Suwanagool, P., Prakasvejakit, S., Leelakusolwong, S., Eampokalap, B., Kachintorn, U., 1996. Causes of chronic diarrhea in patients with AIDS in Thailand: a prospective clinical and microbiological study. J. Gastroenterol. 31, 533–537.

Mansfield, L.S., Gajadhar, A.A., 2004. *Cyclospora cayetanensis*, a food- and waterborne coccidian parasite. Vet. Parasitol. 126, 73–90.

Marangi, M., Koehler, A.V., Zanzani, S.A., Manfredi, M.T., Brianti, E., Giangaspero, A., Gasser, R.B., 2015. Detection of *Cyclospora* in captive chimpanzees and macaques by a quantitative PCR-based mutation scanning approach. Parasit. Vectors 8, 274.

Marder Mph, E.P., Griffin, P.M., Cieslak, P.R., Dunn, J., Hurd, S., Jervis, R., Lathrop, S., Muse, A., Ryan, P., Smith, K., Tobin-D'Angelo, M., Vugia, D.J., Holt, K.G., Wolpert, B.J., Tauxe, R., Geissler, A.L., 2018. Preliminary incidence and trends of infections with pathogens transmitted commonly through food—foodborne diseases active surveillance network, 10 U.S. Sites, 2006-2017. MMWR Morb. Mortal. Wkly Rep. 67, 324–328.

Marek, A., McColl, K., Going, J., Spence, G., Jones, B., Alexander, C., 2012. What a professor learned about Cyclospora cayetanensis by attending Digestive Diseases Week conference in Chicago. Am. J. Gastroenterol. 107, 1109–1111.

Marín-Leonett, M., Figuera, L., Nessi, A., Guzmán, C., Torres, P., Genzlinger, L., Saavedra, G., Ortega, Y.R., 2007. Diarrhea due to Cyclospora-like organism in an immunocompetent patient. J. Infect. Dev. Ctries. 1, 345–347.

Marques, D.F.P., Alexander, C.L., Chalmers, R.M., Elson, R., Freedman, J., Hawkins, G., Lo, J., Robinson, G., Russell, K., Smith-Palmer, A., Kirkbride, H., Chiodini, P., Godbole, G., 2017. Cyclosporiasis in travellers returning to the United Kingdom from Mexico in summer lessons from the recent past to inform the future. Euro Surveill. 22, 30592.

Masucci, L., Graffeo, R., Siciliano, M., Franceschelli, A., Bugli, F., Fadda, G., 2008. First Italian case of cyclosporiasis in an immunocompetent woman: local acquired infection. New Microbiol. 31, 281–284.

Masucci, L., Graffeo, R., Bani, S., Bugli, F., Boccia, S., Nicolotti, N., Fiori, B., Fadda, G., Spanu, T., 2011. Intestinal parasites isolated in a large teaching hospital, Italy, 1 May 2006 to 31 December 2008. Euro Surveill. 16, 19891.

Masuda, G., Ajisawa, A., Imamura, A., Negishi, M., Iseki, M., 2002. Cyclosporiasis: four case reports with a review of the literature. Kansenshogaku Zasshi 76, 416–424 (Article in Japanese).

Mathur, M.K., Verma, A.K., Makwana, G.E., Sinha, M., 2013. Study of opportunistic intestinal parasitic infections in human immunodeficiency virus/acquired immunodeficiency syndrome patients. J. Glob. Infect. 5, 164–167.

McAllister, C.T., Motriuk-Smith, D., Kerr, C.M., 2018. Three new coccidians (Cyclospora, Eimeria) from eastern moles, Scalopus aquaticus (Linnaeus) (Mammalia: Soricomorpha: Talpidae) from Arkansas, USA. Syst. Parasitol. 95, 271–279.

Mendoza, D., Núñez, F.A., Escobedo, A., Pelayo, L., Fernández, M., Torres, D., Cordoví, R.A., 2001. Intestinal parasitic infections in 4 child day-care centers located in San Miguel del Padrón municipality, Havana City, 1998. Rev. Cubana Med. Trop. 53, 189–193 (Article in Spanish).

Milord, F., Lampron-Goulet, E., St-Amour, M., Levac, E., Ramsay, D., 2012. Cyclospora cayetanensis: a description of clinical aspects of an outbreak in Quebec, Canada. Epidemiol. Infect. 140, 626–632.

Mohandas, Sehgal, R., Sud, A., Malla, N., 2002. Prevalence of intestinal parasitic pathogens in HIV-seropositive individuals in Northern India. Jpn. J. Infect. Dis. 55, 83–84.

Morakote, N., Siriprasert, P., Piangjai, S., Vitayasai, P., Tookyang, B., Uparanukraw, P., 1995. Microsporidium and Cyclospora in human stools in Chiang Mai, Thailand. Southeast Asian J. Trop. Med. Public Health 26, 799–800.

Mosimann, M., Nguyen, X.M., Furrer, H., 1999. Excessive watery diarrhea and pronounced fatigue due to Cyclospora cayetanensis infection in an HIV infected traveler returning from the tropics. Schweiz. Med. Wochenschr. 129, 1158–1161 (Article in German).

Mukhopadhyay, C., Wilson, G., Pradhan, D., Shivananda, P.G., 2007. Intestinal protozoal infestation profile in persistent diarrhea in children below age 5 years in western Nepal. Southeast Asian J. Trop. Med. Public Health 38, 13–19.

Naito, T., Mizue, S., Misawa, S., Nakamura, A., Isonuma, H., Kondo, S., Dambara, T., Yamamoto, N., 2009. Cyclospora infection in an immunocompetent patient in Japan. Jpn. J. Infect. Dis. 62, 57–58.

Nassef, N.E., el-Ahl, S.A., el-Shafee, O.K., Nawar, M., 1998. Cyclospora: a newly identified protozoan pathogen of man. J. Egypt. Soc. Parasitol. 28, 213–219.

Nath, J., Hussain, G., Singha, B., Paul, J., Ghosh, S.K., 2015. Burden of major diarrheagenic protozoan parasitic co-infection among amoebic dysentery cases from North East India: a case report. Parasitology 142, 1318–1325.

Nichols, G.L., Freedman, J., Pollock, K.G., Rumble, C., Chalmers, R.M., Chiodini, P., Hawkins, G., Alexander, C.L., Godbole, G., Williams, C., Kirkbride, H.A., Hamel, M., Hawker, J.I., 2015. *Cyclospora* infection linked to travel to Mexico, June to September 2015. Euro Surveill. 20, 30048.

Nimri, L.F., 2003. *Cyclospora cayetanensis* and other intestinal parasites associated with diarrhea in a rural area of Jordan. Int. Microbiol. 6, 131–135.

Nimri, L.F., Meqdam, M., 2004. Enteropathogens associated with cases of gastroenteritis in a rural population in Jordan. Clin. Microbiol. Infect. 10, 634–639.

Nsagha, D.S., Njunda, A.L., Assob, N.J.C., Ayima, C.W., Tanue, E.A., Kibu, O.D., Kwenti, T.E., 2016. Intestinal parasitic infections in relation to CD4(+) T cell counts and diarrhea in HIV/AIDS patients with or without antiretroviral therapy in Cameroon. BMC Infect. Dis. 16, 9.

Nundy, S., Gilman, R.H., Xiao, L., Cabrera, L., Cama, R., Ortega, Y.R., Kahn, G., Cama, V.A., 2011. Wealth and its associations with enteric parasitic infections in a low-income community in Peru: use of principal component analysis. Am. J. Trop. Med. Hyg. 84, 38–42.

Núñez Fernández, F.A., Gálvez Oviedo, M.D., Finlay Villalvilla, C.M., 1995. The first report in Cuba of human intestinal infection by *Cyclospora cayetanensis*, Ortega, 1993. Rev. Cubana. Med. Trop. 47, 211–214 (Article in Spanish).

Núñez, F.A., González, O.M., Bravo, J.R., Escobedo, A.A., González, I., 2003a. Intestinal parasitosis in children admitted to the Pediatric Teaching Hospital of Cerro, Havana City, Cuba. Rev. Cubana Med. Trop. 55, 19–26 (Article in Spanish).

Núñez, F.A., González, O.M., González, I., Escobedo, A.A., Cordoví, R.A., 2003b. Intestinal coccidia in Cuban pediatric patients with diarrhea. Mem. Inst. Oswaldo Cruz 98, 539–542.

Ooi, W.W., Zimmerman, S.K., Needham, C.A., 1995. *Cyclospora* species as a gastrointestinal pathogen in immunocompetent hosts. J. Clin. Microbiol. 33, 1267–1269.

Opoku, Y.K., Boampong, J.N., Ayi, I., Kwakye-Nuako, G., Obiri-Yeboah, D., Koranteng, H., Ghartey-Kwansah, G., Asare, K.K., 2018. Socio-behavioral risk factors associated with cryptosporidiosis in HIV/AIDS patients visiting the HIV referral clinic at cape coast teaching hospital, Ghana. Open AIDS J. 12, 106–116.

Orozco-Mosqueda, G.E., Martínez-Loya, O.A., Ortega, Y.R., 2014. *Cyclospora cayetanensis* in a pediatric hospital in Morelia, México. Am. J. Trop. Med. Hyg. 91, 537–540.

Ortega, Y.R., Sanchez, R., 2010. Update on *Cyclospora cayetanensis*, a food-borne and water-borne parasite. Clin. Microbiol. Rev. 23, 218–234.

Osman, G.A., Makled, K.M., El-Shakankiry, H.M., Metwali, D.M., Abdel-Aziz, S.S., Saafan, H.H., 1999. Coccidian parasites as a cause of watery diarrhoea among protein energy malnourished and other immunocompromised Egyptian children. J. Egypt. Soc. Parasitol. 29, 653–668.

Ozdamar, M., Hakko, E., Turkoglu, S., 2010. High occurrence of cyclosporiasis in Istanbul, Turkey, during a dry and warm summer. Parasit. Vectors 3, 39.

Pandey, P., Bodhidatta, L., Lewis, M., Murphy, H., Shlim, D.R., Cave, W., Rajah, R., Springer, M., Batchelor, T., Sornsakrin, S., Mason, C.J., 2011. Travelers' diarrhea in Nepal: an update on the pathogens and antibiotic resistance. J. Travel Med. 18, 102–108.

Pape, J.W., Verdier, R.I., Boncy, M., Boncy, J., Johnson Jr., W.D., 1994. *Cyclospora* infection in adults infected with HIV. Clinical manifestations, treatment, and prophylaxis. Ann. Intern. Med. 121, 654–657.

Parija, S.C., Bhattacharya, S., Pictorial, C.M.E., 2000. *Isospora belli* and *Cyclospora cayetanensis* in a case of chronic diarrhoea in an immunocompromised host. J. Assoc. Physicians India 48, 1192.

Paschke, C., Apelt, N., Fleischmann, E., Perona, P., Walentiny, C., Löscher, T., Herbinger, K.H., 2011. Controlled study on enteropathogens in travellers returning from the tropics with and without diarrhoea. Clin. Microbiol. Infect. 17, 1194–1200.

Peréz Cordón, G., Cordova Paz Soldan, O., Vargas Vásquez, F., Velasco Soto, J.R., Sempere Bordes, L., Sánchez Moreno, M., Rosales, M.J., 2008. Prevalence of enteroparasites and genotyping of *Giardia lamblia* in Peruvian children. Parasitol. Res. 103, 459–465.

Petry, F., Hofstätter, J., Schulz, B.K., Deitrich, G., Jung, M., Schirmacher, P., 1997. *Cyclospora cayetanensis*: first imported infections in Germany. Infection 25, 167–170.

Pham-Duc, P., Nguyen-Viet, H., Hattendorf, J., Zinsstag, J., Phung-Dac, C., Zurbrügg, C., Odermatt, P., 2013. Ascaris lumbricoides and Trichuris trichiura infections associated with wastewater and human excreta use in agriculture in Vietnam. Parasitol. Int. 62, 172–180.

Pingé-Suttor, V., Douglas, C., Wettstein, A., 2004. *Cyclospora* infection masquerading as coeliac disease. Med. J. Aust. 180, 295–296.

Ponce-Macotela, M., Cob-Sosa, C., Martínez-Gordillo, M.N., 1996. *Cyclospora* in 2 Mexican children. Rev. Invest. Clin. 48, 461–463 (Article in Spanish).

Pons, S., Darles, C., Aguilon, P., Gaillard, T., Brisou, P., 2012. Watery diarrhea in an immune-competent traveler. J. Clin. Microbiol. 50, 3821–3822.

Popovici, I., Dahorea, C., Rugină, A., Coman, G., 2003. Acute diarrhea associated with *Cyclospora cayetanensis*. Rev. Med. Chir. Soc. Med. Nat. Iasi. 107, 877–880 (Article in Romanian).

Portillo, M.E., Pérez-García, A., Fernández-Alonso, M., Rubio, M., 2010. *Cyclospora cayetanensis* in a patient with traveller's diarrhoea. Med. Clin. (Barc.) 134, 377–378 (Article in Spanish).

Pratdesaba, R.A., González, M., Piedrasanta, E., Mérida, C., Contreras, K., Vela, C., Culajay, F., Flores, L., Torres, O., 2001. *Cyclospora cayetanensis* in three populations at risk in Guatemala. J. Clin. Microbiol. 39, 2951–2953.

Puente, S., Morente, A., García-Benayas, T., Subirats, M., Gascón, J., González-Lahoz, J.M., 2006. Cyclosporiasis: a point source outbreak acquired in Guatemala. J. Travel Med. 13, 334–337.

Purych, D.B., Perry, I.L., Bulawka, D., Kowalewska-Grochowska, K.T., Oldale, B.L., 1995. A case of *Cyclospora* infection in an Albertan traveller. Can. Commun. Dis. Rep. 21, 88–91 (Article in English, French).

Rabold, J.G., Hoge, C.W., Shlim, D.R., Kefford, C., Rajah, R., Echeverria, P., 1994. *Cyclospora* outbreak associated with chlorinated drinking water. Lancet 344, 1360–1361.

Raccurt, C.P., Pannier Stockman, C., Eyma, E., Verdier, R.I., Totet, A., Pape, J.W., 2006. Enteric parasites and AIDS in Haiti: utility of detection and treatment of intestinal parasites in family members. Med. Trop. 66, 461–464 (Article in French).

Raccurt, C.P., Fouché, B., Agnamey, P., Menotti, J., Chouaki, T., Totet, A., Pape, J.W., 2008. Presence of *Enterocytozoon bieneusi* associated with intestinal coccidia in patients with chronic diarrhea visiting an HIV center in Haiti. Am. J. Trop. Med. Hyg. 79, 579–580.

Raguin, G., Heyer, F., Rousseau, C., Aerts, J., Desplaces, N., Deluol, A., 1995. *Cyclospora* infection in a HIV infected patient. Presse Med. 24, 1134 (Article in French).

Rai, S.K., Gurung, R., Saiju, R., Bajracharya, L., Rai, N., Gurung, K., Shakya, B., Pant, J., Psharma, Shrestha, A., Rai, C.K., 2008. Intestinal parasitosis among subjects undergoing cataract surgery at the eye camps in rural hilly areas of Nepal. Nepal Med. Coll. J. 10, 100–103.

Ramírez-Olivencia, G., Herrero, M.D., Subirats, M., Rivas González, P., Puente, S., 2008. *Cyclospora cayetanensis* outbreak in travelers to Cuba. Enferm. Infecc. Microbiol. Clin. 26, 558–560 (Article in Spanish).

Rezk, H., el-Shazly, A.M., Soliman, M., el-Nemr, H.I., Nagaty, I.M., Fouad, M.A., 2001. Coccidiosis among immuno-competent and -compromised adults. J. Egypt. Soc. Parasitol. 31, 823–834.

Ribas, A., Jollivet, C., Morand, S., Thongmalayvong, B., Somphavong, S., Siew, C.C., Ting, P.J., Suputtamongkol, S., Saensombath, V., Sanguankiat, S., Tan, B.H., Pa123boune, P., Akkhavong, K., Chaisiri, K., 2017. Intestinal parasitic infections and environmental water contamination in a Rural Village of Northern Lao PDR. Korean J. Parasitol. 55, 523–532.

Ribes, J.A., Seabolt, J.P., Overman, S.B., 2004. Point prevalence of *Cryptosporidium*, *Cyclospora*, and *Isospora* infections in patients being evaluated for diarrhea. Am. J. Clin. Pathol. 122, 28–32.

Richardson Jr., R.F., Remler, B.F., Katirji, B., Murad, M.H., 1998. Guillain-Barré syndrome after *Cyclospora* infection. Muscle Nerve 21, 669–671.

Rivero-Rodríguez, Z., Hernández, A., Bracho, Á., Salazar, S., Villalobos, R., 2013. Prevalence of intestinal microsporidia and other intestinal parasites in hiv positive patients from Maracaibo, Venezuela. Biomedica 33, 538–545 (Article in Spanish).

Rizk, H., Soliman, M., 2001. Coccidiosis among malnourished children in Mansoura, Dakahlia Governorate, Egypt. J. Egypt Soc. Parasitol. 31, 877–886.

Roldán, W.H., Espinoza, Y.A., Huapaya, P.E., Huiza, A.F., Sevilla, C.R., Jiménez, S., 2009. Frequency of human toxocariasis in a rural population from Cajamarca, Peru determined by DOT-ELISA test. Rev. Inst. Med. Trop. Sao Paulo 51, 67–71.

Sakakibara, Y., Takigawa, A., Kawabata, Y., Hirotani, T., Mukai, K., Matsumoto, K., Nakanishi, F., Tanaka, Y., Masuda, E., Hijioka, T., 2010. An imported Japanese case of cyclosporiasis. Nihon Shokakibyo Gakkai Zasshi 107, 1290–1295 (Article in Japanese).

Saksirisampant, W., Prownebon, J., Saksirisampant, P., Mungthin, M., Siripatanapipong, S., Leelayoova, S., 2009. Intestinal parasitic infections: prevalences in HIV/AIDS patients in a Thai AIDS-care centre. Ann. Trop. Med. Parasitol. 103, 573–581.

Samie, A., Guerrant, R.L., Barrett, L., Bessong, P.O., Igumbor, E.O., Obi, C.L., 2009. Prevalence of intestinal parasitic and bacterial pathogens in diarrhoeal and non-diarroeal human stools from Vhembe district, South Africa. J. Health Popul. Nutr. 27, 739–745.

Sancak, B., Akyon, Y., Ergüven, S., 2006. *Cyclospora* infection in five immunocompetent patients in a Turkish university hospital. J. Med. Microbiol. 55, 459–462.

Sánchez-Vega, J.T., Cabrera-Fuentes, H.A., Romero-Olmedo, A.J., Ortiz-Frías, J.L., Sokolina, F., Barreto, G., 2014. *Cyclospora cayetanensis*: this emerging protozoan pathogen in Mexico. Am. J. Trop. Med. Hyg. 90, 351–353.

Sangaré, I., Bamba, S., Cissé, M., Zida, A., Bamogo, R., Sirima, C., Yaméogo, B.K., Sanou, R., Drabo, F., Dabiré, R.K., Guiguemdé, R.T., 2015. Prevalence of intestinal opportunistic parasites infections in the university hospital of Bobo-Dioulasso, Burkina Faso. Infect. Dis. Poverty 4, 32.

Saurabh, K., Nag, V.L., Dash, S., Maurya, A.K., Hada, V., Agrawal, R., Narula, H., Sharma, A., 2017. Spectrum of parasitic infections in patients with diarrhoea attending a tertiary care hospital in Western Rajasthan, India. J. Clin. Diagn. Res. 11, DC01–DC04.

Schubach, T.M., Neves, E.S., Leite, A.C., Araújo, A.Q., de Moura, H., 1997. *Cyclospora cayetanensis* in an asymptomatic patient infected with HIV and HTLV-1. Trans. R. Soc. Trop. Med. Hyg. 91, 175.

Shah, L., MacDougall, L., Ellis, A., Ong, C., Shyng, S., LeBlanc, L., British Columbia Cyclospora Investigation Team, 2009. Challenges of investigating community outbreaks of cyclosporiasis, British Columbia, Canada. Emerg. Infect. Dis. 15, 1286–1288.

Shah, S., Kongre, V., Kumar, V., Bharadwaj, R., 2016. A study of parasitic and bacterial pathogens associated with diarrhea in HIV-positive patients. Cureus. 8, e807.

Shehata, A.I., Hassanein, F., 2015. Intestinal parasitic infections among mentally handicapped individuals in Alexandria, Egypt. Ann. Parasitol. 61, 275–281.

Sherchand, J.B., Cross, J.H., 2001. Emerging pathogen *Cyclospora cayetanensis* infection in Nepal. Southeast Asian J. Trop. Med. Public Health 32, 143–150.

Shields, J.M., Olson, B.H., 2003. *Cyclospora cayetanensis*: a review of an emerging parasitic coccidian. Int. J. Parasitol. 33, 371–391.

Shlim, D.R., Cohen, M.T., Eaton, M., Rajah, R., Long, E.G., Unger, B.L.P., 1991. An alga like organism associated with an outbreak of prolonged diarrhea among foreigners in Nepal. Am. J. Trop. Med. Hyg. 45, 383–389.

Shlim, D.R., Hoge, C.W., Rajah, R., Scott, R.M., Pandy, P., Echeverria, P., 1999. Persistent high risk of diarrhea among foreigners in Nepal during the first 2 years of residence. Clin. Infect. Dis. 29, 613–616.

Sifuentes-Osornio, J., Porras-Cortés, G., Bendall, R.P., Morales-Villarreal, F., Reyes-Terán, G., Ruiz-Palacios, G.M., 1995. Cyclospora cayetanensis infection in patients with and without AIDS: biliary disease as another clinical manifestation. Clin. Infect. Dis. 21, 1092–1097.

Sinniah, B., Rajeswari, B., Johari, S., Ramakrishnan, K., Yusoff, S.W., Rohela, M., 1994. Cyclospora sp. causing diarrhea in man. Southeast Asian J. Trop. Med. Public Health 25, 221–223.

Siripanth, C., Phraevanich, R., Suphadtanaphongs, W., Thima, N., Radomyos, P., 2002. Cyclospora cayetanensis: oocyst characteristics and excystation. Southeast Asian J. Trop. Med. Public Health 33, 45–48.

Smith, H.V., Paton, C.A., Girdwood, R.W., Mtambo, M.M., 1996. Cyclospora in non-human primates in Gombe. Vet. Rec. 138, 528.

Stewart, W.C., Pollock, K.G., Browning, L.M., Young, D., Smith-Palmer, A., Reilly, W.J., 2005. Survey of zoonoses recorded in Scotland between 1993 and 2002. Vet. Rec. 157, 697–702.

Swarna, S.R., Madhavan, R., Gomathi, S., Yadav, D., 2013. Chronic diarrhea due to Cyclospora spp. infection. Trop. Parasitol. 3, 85–86.

Swathirajan, C.R., Vignesh, R., Pradeep, A., Solomon, S.S., Solomon, S., Balakrishnan, P., 2017. Occurrence of enteric parasitic infections among HIV-infected individuals and its relation to CD4 T-cell counts with a special emphasis on coccidian parasites at a tertiary care centre in South India. Indian J. Med. Microbiol. 35, 37–40.

Tandukar, S., Ansari, S., Adhikari, N., Shrestha, A., Gautam, J., Sharma, B., Rajbhandari, D., Gautam, S., Nepal, H.P., Sherchand, J.B., 2013. Intestinal parasitosis in school children of Lalitpur district of Nepal. BMC. Res. Notes 6, 449.

Taş Cengiz, Z., Beyhan, Y.E., Yılmaz, H., 2016. Cyclospora cayetanensis, opportunistic protozoan parasite, in Van Province, Turkey: a report of seven cases. Turkiye Parazitol. Derg. 40, 166–168.

Thima, K., Mori, H., Praevanit, R., Mongkhonmu, S., Waikagul, J., Watthanakulpanich, D., 2014. Recovery of Cyclospora cayetanensis among asymptomatic rural Thai schoolchildren. Asian Pac. J. Trop. Med. 7, 119–123.

Tiwari, B.R., Ghimire, P., Malla, S., Sharma, B., Karki, S., 2013. Intestinal parasitic infection among the HIV-infected patients in Nepal. J. Infect. Dev. Ctries. 7, 550–555.

Torres-Slimming, P.A., Mundaca, C.C., Moran, M., Quispe, J., Colina, O., Bacon, D.J., Lescano, A.G., Gilman, R.H., Blazes, D.L., 2006. Outbreak of cyclosporiasis at a naval base in Lima, Peru. Am. J. Trop. Med. Hyg. 75, 546–548.

Tsang, O.T., Wong, R.W., Lam, B.H., Chan, J.M., Tsang, K.Y., Leung, W.S., 2013. Cyclospora infection in a young woman with human immunodeficiency virus in Hong Kong: a case report. BMC. Res. Notes 6, 521.

Tuli, L., Gulati, A.K., Sundar, S., Mohapatra, T.M., 2008. Correlation between CD4 counts of HIV patients and enteric protozoan in different seasons—an experience of a tertiary care hospital in Varanasi (India). BMC Gastroenterol. 8, 36.

Tuli, L., Singh, D.K., Gulati, A.K., Sundar, S., Mohapatra, T.M., 2010. A multiattribute utility evaluation of different methods for the detection of enteric protozoa causing diarrhea in AIDS patients. BMC Microbiol. 10, 11.

Turgay, N., Yolasiğmaz, A., Uner, A., 2006. A human case of cyclosporiasis after traveling in the subtropics. Turkiye Parazitol. Derg. 30, 83–85 (Article in Turkish).

Turgay, N., Yolasigmaz, A., Erdogan, D.D., Zeyrek, F.Y., Uner, A., 2007. Incidence of cyclosporiasis in patients with gastrointestinal symptoms in western Turkey. Med. Sci. Monit. 13, CR34–39.

Turgay, N., Unver-Yolasığmaz, A., Oyur, T., Bardak-Özcem, S., Töz, S., 2012. Monthly distribution of intestinal parasites detected in a part of western Turkey between May 2009-April 2010-results of acid fast and modified trichrome staining methods. Turkiye Parazitol. Derg. 36, 71–74 (Article in Turkish).

Türk, M., Türker, M., Ak, M., Karaayak, B., Kaya, T., 2004. Cyclosporiasis associated with diarrhoea in an immunocompetent patient in Turkey. J. Med. Microbiol. 53, 255–257.

Uga, S., Kimura, D., Kimura, K., Margono, S.S., 2002. Intestinal parasitic infections in Bekasi district, West Java, Indonesia and a comparison of the infection rates determined by different techniques for fecal examination. Southeast Asian J. Trop. Med. Public Health 33, 462–467.

Uysal, H.K., Adas, G.T., Atalik, K., Altiparmak, S., Akgul, O., Saribas, S., Gurcan, M., Yuksel, P., Yildirmak, T., Kocazeybek, B., Ziver, T., Oner, Y.A., 2017. The prevalence of *Cyclospora cayetanensis* and *Cryptosporidium* spp. in Turkish patients infected with HIV-1. Acta Parasitol. 62, 557–564.

van Gool, T., Dankert, J., 1996. 3 emerging protozoal infections in The Netherlands: *Cyclospora, Dientamoeba*, and *Microspora* infections. Ned. Tijdschr. Geneeskd. 140, 155–160 (Article in Dutch).

Varma, M., Hester, J.D., Schaefer 3rd, F.W., Ware, M.W., Lindquist, H.D., 2003. Detection of *Cyclospora cayetanensis* using a quantitative real-time PCR assay. J. Microbiol. Methods 53, 27–36.

Vásquez, T.O., Alvarez Ch, R., Gonzales, S.N., Neme, D.G.A., Romero, C.R., Valencia, R.S., Gomez, A.V., Martinez, B.I., 1998. Diagnosis and treatment of *cyclospora cayetanensis* infection in paediatric patients. Rev. Gastroenterol. Peru. 18, 116–120 (Article in Spanish).

Velásquez, J.N., Carnevale, S., Cabrera, M., Kuo, L., Chertcoff, A., Mariano, M., Bozzini, J.P., Etchart, C., Argento, R., di Risio, C., 2004. *Cyclospora cayetanensis* in patients with AIDS and chronic diarrhea. Acta Gastroenterol. Latinoam. 34, 133–137 (Article in Spanish).

Verdier, R.I., Fitzgerald, D.W., Johnson Jr., W.D., Pape, J.W., 2000. Trimethoprim-sulfamethoxazole compared with ciprofloxacin for treatment and prophylaxis of Isospora belli and *Cyclospora cayetanensis* infection in HIV-infected patients. A randomized, controlled trial. Ann. Intern. Med. 132, 885–888.

Viriyavejakul, P., Nintasen, R., Punsawad, C., Chaisri, U., Punpoowong, B., Riganti, M., 2009. High prevalence of microsporidium infection in HIV-infected patients. Southeast Asian J. Trop. Med. Public Health 40, 223–228.

Visvesvara, G.S., Arrowood, M.J., Qvarnstrom, Y., Sriram, R., Bandea, R., Wilkins, P.P., Farnon, E., Weitzman, G., 2013. Concurrent parasitic infections in a renal transplant patient. Emerg. Infect. Dis. 19, 2044–2045.

Wanachiwanawin, D., Lertlaituan, P., Manatsathit, S., Tunsupasawasdikul, S., Suwanagool, P., Thakerngpol, K., 1995. *Cyclospora* infection in an HIV infected patient with ultrastructural study. Southeast Asian J. Trop. Med. Public Health 26, 375–377.

Wang, K.X., Li, C.P., Wang, J., Tian, Y., 2002. *Cyclospore cayetanensis* in Anhui, China. World J. Gastroenterol. 8, 1144–1148.

Weitz, J.C., Weitz, C.R., Canales, M.R., Moya, R.R., 2009. *Cyclospora cayetanensis* infection: updated review a propos of three cases of traveler's diarrhea. Rev. Chilena. Infectol. 26, 549–554 (Article in Spanish).

Whitfield, Y., Johnson, K., Hanson, H., Huneault, D., 2015. Outbreak of Cyclosporiasis linked to the consumption of imported sugar snap peas in Ontario, Canada. J. Food Prot. 80, 1666–1669.

Wiwanitkit, V., 2006. Intestinal parasite infestation in HIV infected patients. Curr. HIV Res. 4, 87–96.

Xiao, S.M., Li, G.Q., Zhou, R.Q., Li, W.H., Yang, J.W., 2007. Combined PCR-oligonucleotide ligation assay for detection of dairy cattle-derived *Cyclospora* sp. Vet. Parasitol. 149, 185–190.

Yadav, P., Khalil, S., Mirdha, B.R., Makharia, G.K., Bhatnagar, S., 2015. Molecular characterization of clinical isolates of *Cyclospora cayetanensis* from patients with diarrhea in India. Indian J. Med. Microbiol. 33, 351–356.

Yadav, P., Khalil, S., Mirdha, B.R., 2016. Molecular appraisal of intestinal parasitic infection in transplant recipients. Indian J. Med. Res. 144, 258–263.

Yai, L.E., Bauab, A.R., Hirschfeld, M.P., de Oliveira, M.L., Damaceno, J.T., 1997. The first two cases of *Cyclospora* in dogs, São Paulo, Brazil. Rev. Inst. Med. Trop. Sao Paulo 39, 177–179.

Yamada, M., Hatama, S., Ishikawa, Y., Kadota, K., 2014. Intranuclear coccidiosis caused by *Cyclospora* spp. in calves. J. Vet. Diagn. Invest. 26, 678–682.

Yazar, S., Yaman, O., Demirtaş, F., Yalçin, S., Yücesoy, M., Sahin, I., 2002. *Cyclospora cayetanensis* associated with diarrhea in a patient with idiopathic compensated hepatic cirrhosis. Acta Gastroenterol. Belg. 65, 241–244.

Yazar, S., Yalcln, S., Sahin, I., 2004. Human *cyclosporiosis* in Turkey. World J. Gastroenterol. 10, 1844–1847.

Yazar, S., Mistik, S., Yaman, O., Yildiz, O., Ozcan, H., Sahin, I., 2009. Three diarrheal cases caused by *Cyclospora* cayetanensis in Kayseri. Turkiye Parazitol. Derg. 33, 85–88 (Article in Turkish).

Ye, J., Xiao, L., Li, J., Huang, W., Amer, S.E., Guo, Y., Roellig, D., Feng, Y., 2014. Occurrence of human-pathogenic *Enterocytozoon bieneusi*, *Giardia duodenalis* and *Cryptosporidium* genotypes in laboratory macaques in Guangxi, China. Parasitol. Int. 63, 132–137.

Yılmaz, H., Taş-Cengiz, Z., Ceylan, A., Ekici, A., 2012. The distribution of intestinal parasites in people admitted to the Yüzüncü Yıl University Parasitology Laboratory of Health Research and Training Hospital, in 2009. Turkiye Parazitol. Derg. 36, 105–108 (Article in Turkish).

Yu, J.R., Sohn, W.M., 2003. A case of human cyclosporiasis causing traveler's diarrhea after visiting Indonesia. J. Korean Med. Sci. 18, 738–741.

Zeng, H.H., Huang, M.J., Meng, F.Y., 2005. A case of chronic diarrhea and hypoproteinemia associated with *Cryptosporidium parvum* and *Cyclospora cayetanensis*. Zhonghua Er Ke Za Zhi 43, 797–798 (Article in Chinese).

Zhang, B.X., 2000. A case with *Cyclospora* cayetanensis infection. Zhongguo Ji Sheng Chong Xue Yu Ji Sheng Chong Bing Za Zhi 18, 319 (Article in Chinese).

Zhang, B.X., Yu, H., Zhang, L.L., Tao, H., Li, Y.Z., Li, Y., Cao, Z.K., Bai, Z.M., He, Y.Q., 2002. Prevalence survey on *Cyclospora cayetanensis* and *Cryptosporidium* ssp. in diarrhea cases in Yunnan Province. Zhongguo Ji Sheng Chong Xue Yu Ji Sheng Chong Bing Za Zhi 20, 106–108 (Article in Chinese).

Zhao, G.H., Cong, M.M., Bian, Q.Q., Cheng, W.Y., Wang, R.J., Qi, M., Zhang, L.X., Lin, Q., Zhu, X.Q., 2013. Molecular characterization of *Cyclospora*-like organisms from golden snub-nosed monkeys in Qinling Mountain in Shaanxi province, northwestern China. PLoS ONE 8, e58216.

Zhou, Y., Lv, B., Wang, Q., Wang, R., Jian, F., Zhang, L., Ning, C., Fu, K., Wang, Y., Qi, M., Yao, H., Zhao, J., Zhang, X., Sun, Y., Shi, K., Arrowood, M.J., Xiao, L., 2011. Prevalence and molecular characterization of *Cyclospora cayetanensis*, Henan, China. Emerg. Infect. Dis. 17, 1887–1890.

CHAPTER 5

Transmission risk factors

Contents

5.1 Introduction

Human cyclosporiasis is caused by *Cyclospora cayetanensis*, and it typically induced periodic profuse watery diarrhea (Shields and Olson, 2003; Ortega and Sanchez, 2010; Almeria et al., 2019; Giangaspero and Gasser, 2019). Human *C. cayetanensis* infection has been documented in over 56 countries worldwide, and 13 of these have recorded cyclosporiasis outbreaks (Li et al., 2020). The latest large scale of cyclosporiasis outbreaks occurred in 2013 and 2018 in multiple states of the United States (Abanyie et al., 2015; Casillas et al., 2018).

In humans, most of these infections are contracted via the fecal-oral route, and water, berries, basil, cilantro, and other food produce can be a vehicle for *Cyclospora* transmission (Almeria et al., 2019). The *Cyclospora* infection is evidenced to be linked with the consumption of contaminated food and water or contact with transmission vehicles of oocysts (Li et al., 2020).

Many large cyclosporiasis outbreaks have been documented in industrialized nations (Ortega and Sanchez, 2010). Among them, food has been identified as the main vehicle for *Cyclospora* transmission, according to source tracing studies (Herwaldt and Ackers, 1997; Ortega and Sanchez, 2010). Cilantro from Mexico was identified as one of the potential sources of cyclosporiasis outbreak in the United States (US) in 2013, with more than 600 cases of infection (Abanyie et al., 2015). Prepackaged vegetable trays and vegetable salads sold at a fast food chain were suspected as the

Cyclospora and Cyclosporiasis
https://doi.org/10.1016/B978-0-12-821616-3.00007-2

sources of another cyclosporiasis outbreak during the June and July of 2018 by trace-back investigations (Casillas et al., 2018).

Several large outbreaks of cyclosporiasis had been reported in the world (Li et al., 2020). Although large outbreaks of cyclosporiasis have been mainly documented in developed countries, *C. cayetanensis* infections are most commonly reported in developing countries or in endemic areas (Li et al., 2020). In susceptible individuals, cyclosporiasis is reported to be most prevalent in immunocompetent diarrheic patients (Li et al., 2020). There are notable seasonal distributions of *C. cayetanensis* infections that commonly occur in rainy or summer season (Zhou et al., 2011; Kaminsky et al., 2016). Cyclosporiasis causes significant health problem to the people traveling or expatriating to the under developed or developing countries having poor sanitation and high population density (Fryauff et al., 1999; Mansfield and Gajadhar, 2004; Pandey et al., 2011; Kłudkowska et al., 2017).

5.2 Marked seasonality transmissions

Marked seasonality (rainy season or summer) has been observed in human *C. cayetanensis* infection in the Northern Hemisphere, including China (Zhou et al., 2011; Jiang et al., 2018), Nepal (Sherchand and Cross, 2001; Kimura et al., 2005; Bhandari et al., 2015), Turkey (Ozdamar et al., 2010), Honduras (Kaminsky et al., 2016), and Mexico (Orozco-Mosqueda et al., 2014). The consistent pattern of seasonal distribution is likely indicative of optimal environmental conditions (temperature and humidity) that are required for oocysts to sporulate.

5.3 Animal reservoirs

Several *Cyclospora* species or *Cyclospora*-like organisms have been reported in various animals (Table 5.1), including five *Cyclospora* species identified in primates (Eberhard et al., 1999a, b; Eberhard et al., 2001a, b; Ortega and Sanchez, 2010; Li et al., 2015). *Cyclospora*-like organisms have been documented in dogs, cattle, chickens, rats/house mice, birds, and even shellfish. The Asian freshwater clams (*Corbicula fluminea*) can recover oocysts of *C. cayetanensis* by artificial infection contamination, thus could be used as a biological indicator of water contamination with oocysts (Graczyk et al., 1998). In one study in Nepal, the households keeping livestock had higher *Cyclospora* infection rates (Bhandari et al., 2015).

Table 5.1 *Cyclospora* spp. or *Cyclospora*-like organisms were reported in various animals.

Countries (site)	Host	Sample number	Positive number	Prevalence	Detection methods	References
Brazil, São Paulo	Dogs		2 cases		PCR–RFLP identify	Yai et al. (1997)
China, Guangzhou	Dairy cattle		2 cases		PCR–OLA identify	Li et al. (2007)
China	Dairy cattle	168	6	3.57%	PCR identify	Xiao et al. (2007)
China, Shaanxi	Golden snub-nosed monkeys	71	2	2.82%	PCR identify	Zhao et al. (2013)
China, Guangxi	Crab-eating macaques	205	1	0.49%	PCR identify	Ye et al. (2014)
China, Guizhou	Rhesus monkeys	411	28	6.81%	PCR identify	Li et al. (2015)
China	Monkeys	3349	7	0.21%	Light microscopy	Li et al. (2017)
Egypt	Dogs	130	1	0.77%	Light microscopy	Awadallah and Salem (2015)
Equatorial Guinea	Drills (*Mandrillus leucophaeus poensis*)	51	11	21.57%	PCR identify	Eberhard et al. (2014)
Ethiopia	Baboons	59	8	13.56%	Modified Ziehl–Neelsen satin	Legesse and Erko (2004)
Ethiopia	Vervet monkeys	41	9	21.95%	Modified Ziehl–Neelsen satin	Legesse and Erko (2004)
India	Sheep	65	2	3.08%	Ziehl-Neelsen stain and confirmed with PCR	Basnett et al. (2018)
India	Goat	216	4	1.85%	Ziehl-Neelsen stain and confirmed with PCR	Basnett et al. (2018)
Italy	Monkeys	119	11	9.24%	qPCR identify	Marangi et al. (2015)
Japan	Claves		3 cases		PCR identify	Yamada et al. (2014)
Kenya	No-human primates	511	81	15.85%	PCR identify	Eberhard et al. (2001a, b)
Kenya	Baboons	235	42	17.87%	PCR identify	Li et al. (2011)

Continued

Table 5.1 Cyclospora spp. or Cyclospora-like organisms were reported in various animals.—cont'd

Countries (site)	Host	Sample number	Positive number	Prevalence	Detection methods	References
Malaysia	Large-billed crow	106	6	5.66%	Modified Ziehl–Neelsen satin	Lee et al. (2008)
Mexico	Chicken		1 case		Kinyoun's acid-fast stain; autofluorescence under UV	García-López et al. (1996)
Nepal	Chicken	110	3	2.73%		Sherchand and Cross (2001)
Nepal	Dogs	90	2	2.22%		Sherchand and Cross (2001)
Nepal	Rats/House mice	50	2	4.00%		Sherchand and Cross (2001)
Nepal	Dog	14	2	14.29%	PCR identify	Chu et al. (2004)
Nepal	Chicken	3	1	33.33%	PCR identify	Chu et al. (2004)
Nepal	Monkey	3	1	33.33%	PCR identify	Chu et al. (2004)
Spain	Birds	984	23	2.34%	Harada–Mori technique satin	Cordón et al. (2008)
Spain	No-human primates	18	6	33.33%	Modified Ziehl–Neelsen satin	Cordón et al. (2008)
Spain	Carnivora animals	72	3	4.17%	Modified Ziehl–Neelsen satin	Cordón et al. (2008)
Spain	Artiodactyla animals	198	18	9.09%	Modified Ziehl–Neelsen satin	Cordón et al. (2008)
Thailand, Samutprakarn	Cockroaches	920	10	1.09%	Modified acid-fast stain	Chamavit et al. (2011)
Tanzania	Baboons		3 cases		PCR identify	Smith et al. (1996)
Tunisia	Wild shellfish	1255	526	41.91%	qPCR identify	Ghozzi et al. (2017)
Turkey (Bays of Izmir and Mersin)	Edible shellfish	53	14	26.42%	qPCR/HRM identify	Aksoy et al. (2014)
US	Howler monkey	96	17	17.71%		Helenbrook et al. (2015)
Total		9603	847	8.82%		

Another study attempted to develop an animal model for *C. cayetanensis* to study human cyclosporiasis. Various types of animal (various strains of mice, rats, sand rats, chickens, ducks, rabbits, birds, hamsters, ferrets, pigs, dogs, owl monkeys, rhesus monkeys, and cynomolgus monkeys) were inoculated with human *C. cayetanensis* oocysts by gavage. None of the animals developed patent infection or signs of infection 4–6 weeks after inoculation. It was concluded that none of the mammals tested are susceptible to infection with *C. cayetanensis* (Graczyk et al., 1998).

A pilot study sought to infect human volunteers with *C. cayetanensis*; however, no oocysts were detected in any stool samples during the 16-week trial in any of the seven volunteers (Alfano-Sobsey et al., 2004). Given the results of this study, the conditions necessary for *Cyclospora* to become infectious were likely not maintained when preparing or storing the oocysts. Further studies are necessary to assess the effects of temperature, humidity, storage conditions, and disinfection on the survival, viability, and infectivity of stored *Cyclospora* oocysts.

5.4 Food/water/soil sample contamination

In industrialized countries or regions, cyclosporiasis has most often been linked to foodborne outbreaks (Rose and Slifko, 1999). In developing countries or endemic areas, recorded *C. cayetanensis* infections have been related to contact with contaminated food, water, or soil (Burstein Alva, 2005; Chacín-Bonilla, 2008a, b; Bhandari et al., 2015). In a community in Venezuela, a strong association between environmental contact with fecal-contaminated soil and cyclosporiasis occurrence was found, suggesting that contact with soil may be an important mode of transmission (Chacín-Bonilla, 2008a, b).

There are many records of vegetables, fruits, water, or soil being contaminated with *Cyclospora* oocysts in countries as diverse as Italy (Giangaspero et al., 2015), Malaysia (Bilung et al., 2017), Peru (Sturbaum et al., 1998), Nepal (Sherchand and Cross, 2001), and Vietnam (Tram et al., 2008), among others (Table 5.2). As well as, numerous methods have been developed for the recovery and analysis of *Cyclospora* oocysts in contaminated food, water, and soil samples (Robertson et al., 2000; Shields et al., 2012).

Due to recent outbreaks of cyclosporiasis associated with the consumption of fresh produces (Li et al., 2020), producers are demanding modern microbiological tools for the rapid and accurate identification of the human pathogen *C. cayetanensis* in fresh food and environmental samples.

Table 5.2 *Cyclospora* spp. or *Cyclospora*-like organisms were reported in water, soil or produce vehicle.

Country (site)	Source	Sample number	Positive number	Prevalence	Detection methods	References
Water or soil						
Cambodia, Phnom Penh	Water spinach	36	3	8.33%	Standard methods	Vuong et al. (2007)
Egypt, Dakahli	Potable water samples	840	2	0.24%	Modified Ziehl-Neelsen satin	Elshazly et al. (2007)
Egypt, El-Minia	Water samples	336	40	11.90%	Direct microscopy and modified Ziehl-Neelsen satin	Khalifa et al. (2014)
Ghana, Accra	Sachet water samples	27	16	59.26%	Modified Ziehl-Neelsen satin	Kwakye-Nuako et al. (2007)
Italy, Apulia	Treated water	94	20	21.28%	qPCR-SSCP identify	Giangaspero et al. (2015)
Italy, Apulia	Well water	16	1	6.25%	qPCR-SSCP identify	Giangaspero et al. (2015)
Italy, Apulia	Drinking water	3	0	0	qPCR-SSCP identify	Giangaspero et al. (2015)
Italy, Apulia	Soil	51	6	11.76%	qPCR-SSCP identify	Giangaspero et al. (2015)
Italy	Toilets water samples	3	3	100%	RT-PCR identify	Giangaspero et al. (2015)
Malaysia, Sarawak	Water for recreational activities	12	2	16.67%	Modiied Ziehl-Neelsen satin	Bilung et al. (2017)
Malaysia, Sarawak	Environmental water	24	2	8.33%	Modified Ziehl-Neelsen satin	Bilung et al. (2017)
Nepal	Sewage water		3 cases		Direct microscopic and modified acid fast stain	Sherchand and Cross (2001)
Peru	Wastewater[a]		11 cases		Fluorescent microscopy and PCR	Sturbaum et al. (1998)

Location	Sample	Total	Cases positive	%	Method	Reference
Spain, Madrid	Water Sources	223	20	8.97%	Kinyoun stain and PCR	Galván et al. (2013)
Turkey, Samsun	Water samples	228	56	24.56%	Kinyoun acid-fast, modified trichrome, and trichrome satin	Karaman et al. (2017)
Tunisia	Wastewater and sludge samples	232	1	0.43%	PCR identify	Ben Ayed et al. (2012)
Vietnam, Hanoi	Market water	48	6	12.50%	Before the rainy season	Tram et al. (2008)
Vietnam, Hanoi	Farm water	47	6	12.77%	Before the rainy season	Tram et al. (2008)
US, Texas	Water for drinking	12	5	41.67%	PCR identify	Dowd et al. (2003)
US, Arizona	Influent and effluent wastewater	Cases	positive		Newly developed qPCR identify	Kitajima et al. (2014)
Subtotal		2232	189	8.47%		
Food						
Canada, Ontario	Ready-to-eat packaged leafy greens	544	9	1.65%	PCR-RFLP identify	Dixon et al. (2013)
Egypt	Commercial fresh juices			14.50%	Modified Ziehl-Neelsen stain	Mossallam (2010)
Ethiopia, Jimma	Fruits and vegetables	360	18	5.00%	Modied Zeihl-Neelsen stain	Tefera et al. (2014)
Ghana, Accra	Raw vegetables	168	20	11.90%	Ziehl-Neelsen stain	Duedu et al. (2014)
Italy, Apulia	Vegetables	49	6	12.22%	qPCR-SSCP	Giangaspero et al. (2015)
Italy	Ready-to-eat packaged salads	648	8	1.23%	Microscopy and qPCR identify	Caradonna et al. (2017)
Korea	Vegetables	404	5	1.23%	Multiplex qPCR identify	Sim et al. (2017)

Continued

Table 5.2 *Cyclospora* spp. or *Cyclospora*-like organisms were reported in water, soil or produce vehicle—cont'd

Country (site)	Source	Sample number	Positive number	Prevalence	Detection methods	References
Nepal	Cabbage		3 cases		Direct microscopic and modified acid–fast stain	Sherchand and Cross (2001)
Nepal	Lettuce		2 cases		Direct microscopic and modified acid–fast stain	Sherchand and Cross (2001)
Nepal	Mustard leaves		1 cases		Direct microscopic and modified acid–fast stain	Sherchand and Cross (2001)
Peru	Vegetables			1.80%		Ortega et al. (1997)
Vietnam, Hanoi	Market herb samples	240	28	11.67%	Before the rainy season	Tram et al. (2008)
Vietnam, Hanoi	Farm herb samples	240	22	9.17%	Before the rainy season	Tram et al. (2008)
Subtotal		2653	116	4.37%		

[a]First report in wastewater.

It developed many kinds of molecular tool for the rapid and accurate detection of *C. cayetanensis*, such as in fresh berries based on 18S rRNA gene (Resendiz-Nava et al., 2020) and the internal transcribed spacer 1 (ITS-1) region (Temesgen et al., 2019).

5.5 Conclusions

There are notable seasonal distributions of *C. cayetanensis* infections that commonly occur in rainy or summer season. Although large outbreaks of cyclosporiasis have been mainly documented in developed countries, *C. cayetanensis* infections are most commonly reported in developing countries or in endemic areas. In susceptible individuals, cyclosporiasis is reported to be most prevalent in immunocompetent diarrheic patients. Cyclosporiasis causes significant health problem to the people traveling or expatriating to the under developed or developing countries having poor sanitation and high population density. Consumption or contact with oocysts in contaminated food, water, or soil; contact with animals; and poor sanitation are likely major risk factors for *Cyclospora* transmission. In humans, most of these infections are contracted via the fecal-oral route, and water, berries, basil, cilantro, and other food produce can be a vehicle for *Cyclospora* transmission (Table 5.3).

Table 5.3 Epidemiological determinants and risk factors for human cyclosporiasis.

Factors	Main points
Sources of transmission Cocysts	Suitable environmental temperature and humidity (rainy or summer season)
	Infectious (sporulated) *Cyclospora cayetanensis* oocysts
Routes of transmission Vectors or vehicle	Produce (fresh vegetables or fruits) as the vehicle
	Travel to or residence in endemic areas
	Water/soil as the vehicle
	Poor sanitary conditions
Susceptible human populations	Residents in low-income communities or endemic areas
	Patients with diarrhea or gastroenteritis symptoms
	Immunodeficient patients with diarrhea
	Immunodeficient patients

References

Abanyie, F., Harvey, R.R., Harris, J.R., Wiegand, R.E., Gaul, L., Desvignes-Kendrick, M., Irvin, K., Williams, I., Hall, R.L., Herwaldt, B., Gray, E.B., Qvarnstrom, Y., Wise, M.E., Cantu, V., Cantey, P.T., Bosch, S., da Silva, A.J., Fields, A., Bishop, H., Wellman, A., Beal, J., Wilson, N., Fiore, A.E., Tauxe, R., Lance, S., Slutsker, L., Parise, M., Multistate Cyclosporiasis Outbreak Investigation Team, 2015. 2013 multistate outbreaks of *Cyclospora cayetanensis* infections associated with fresh produce: focus on the Texas investigations. Epidemiol. Infect. 143, 3451–3458.

Aksoy, U., Marangi, M., Papini, R., Ozkoc, S., Bayram Delibas, S., Giangaspero, A., 2014. Detection of *Toxoplasma gondii* and *Cyclospora cayetanensis* in Mytilus galloprovincialis from Izmir Province coast (Turkey) by real time PCR/high-resolution melting analysis (HRM). Food Microbiol. 44, 128–135.

Alfano-Sobsey, E.M., Eberhard, M.L., Seed, J.R., Weber, D.J., Won, K.Y., Nace, E.K., Moe, C.L., 2004. Human challenge pilot study with *Cyclospora cayetanensis*. Emerg. Infect. Dis. 10, 726–728.

Almeria, S., Cinar, H.N., Dubey, J.P., 2019. *Cyclospora cayetanensis* and cyclosporiasis: an update. Microorganisms 7, 317.

Awadallah, M.A., Salem, L.M., 2015. Zoonotic enteric parasites transmitted from dogs in Egypt with special concern to *Toxocara canis* infection. Vet. World 8, 946–957.

Basnett, K., Nagarajan, K., Soundararajan, C., Vairamuthu, S., Sudhakar Rao, G.V., 2018. Morphological and molecular identification of *Cyclospora* species in sheep and goat at Tamil Nadu, India. J. Parasit. Dis. 42, 604–607.

Ben Ayed, L., Yang, W., Widmer, G., Cama, V., Ortega, Y., Xiao, L., 2012. Survey and genetic characterization of wastewater in Tunisia for *Cryptosporidium* spp., *Giardia duodenalis*, *Enterocytozoon bieneusi*, *Cyclospora cayetanensis* and *Eimeria* spp. J. Water Health 10, 431–444.

Bhandari, D., Tandukar, S., Parajuli, H., Thapa, P., Chaudhary, P., Shrestha, D., Shah, P.K., Sherchan, J.B., Sherchand, J.B., 2015. *Cyclospora* infection among school children in Kathmandu, Nepal: prevalence and associated risk factors. Trop. Med. Health 43, 211–216.

Bilung, L.M., Tahar, A.S., Yunos, N.E., Apun, K., Lim, Y.A., Nillian, E., Hashim, H.F., 2017. Detection of *Cryptosporidium* and *Cyclospora* oocysts from environmental water for drinking and recreational activities in Sarawak, Malaysia. Biomed. Res. Int. 2017, 4636420.

Burstein Alva, S., 2005. Cyclosporosis: an emergent parasitosis. (I) Clinical and epidemiological aspects. Rev. Gastroenterol. Peru 25, 328–335.

Caradonna, T., Marangi, M., Del Chierico, F., Ferrari, N., Reddel, S., Bracaglia, G., Normanno, G., Putignani, L., Giangaspero, A., 2017. Detection and prevalence of protozoan parasites in ready-to-eat packaged salads on sale in Italy. Food Microbiol. 67, 67–75.

Casillas, S.M., Bennett, C., Straily, A., 2018. Notes from the field: multiple cyclosporiasis outbreaks—United States, 2018. MMWR Morb. Mortal. Wkly Rep. 67, 1101–1102.

Chacín-Bonilla, L., 2008a. Transmission of *Cyclospora cayetanensis* infection: a review focusing on soil-borne cyclosporiasis. Trans. R. Soc. Trop. Med. Hyg. 102, 215–216.

Chacín-Bonilla, L., 2008b. Transmission of *Cyclospora cayetanensis* infection: a review focusing on soil-borne cyclosporiasis. Trans. R. Soc. Trop. Med. Hyg. 102, 215–216.

Chamavit, P., Sahaisook, P., Niamnuy, N., 2011. The majority of cockroaches from the Samutprakarn province of Thailand are carriers of parasitic organisms. EXCLI J. 10, 218–222.

Chu, D.M., Sherchand, J.B., Cross, J.H., Orlandi, P.A., 2004. Detection of *Cyclospora cayetanensis* in animal fecal isolates from Nepal using an FTA filter-base polymerase chain reaction method. Am. J. Trop. Med. Hyg. 71, 373–379.

Cordón, G.P., Prados, A.H., Romero, D., Moreno, M.S., Pontes, A., Osuna, A., Rosales, M.J., 2008. Intestinal parasitism in the animals of the zoological garden "Peña Escrita" (Almuñecar, Spain). Vet. Parasitol. 156, 302–309.

Dixon, B., Parrington, L., Cook, A., Pollari, F., Farber, J., 2013. Detection of *Cyclospora*, *Cryptosporidium*, and *Giardia* in ready-to-eat packaged leafy greens in Ontario, Canada. J. Food Prot. 76, 307–313.

Dowd, S.E., John, D., Eliopolus, J., Gerba, C.P., Naranjo, J., Klein, R., López, B., de Mejía, M., Mendoza, C.E., Pepper, I.L., 2003. Confirmed detection of *Cyclospora cayetanesis*, *Encephalitozoon intestinalis* and *Cryptosporidium parvum* in water used for drinking. J. Water Health 1, 117–123.

Duedu, K.O., Yarnie, E.A., Tetteh-Quarcoo, P.B., Attah, S.K., Donkor, E.S., Ayeh-Kumi, P.F., 2014. A comparative survey of the prevalence of human parasites found in fresh vegetables sold in supermarkets and open-aired markets in Accra, Ghana. BMC Res. Notes 7, 836.

Eberhard, M.L., da Silva, A.J., Lilley, B.G., Pieniazek, N.J., 1999a. Morphologic and molecular characterization of new *Cyclospora* species from Ethiopian monkeys: *C. cercopitheci* sp.n., *C. colobi* sp.n., and *C. papionis* sp.n. Emerg. Infect. Dis. 5, 651–658.

Eberhard, M.L., da Silva, A.J., Lilley, B.G., Pieniazek, N.J., 1999b. Morphologic and molecular characterization of new *Cyclospora* species from Ethiopian monkeys: *C. cercopitheci* sp.n., *C. colobi* sp.n., and *C. papionis* sp.n. Emerg. Infect. Dis. 5, 651–658.

Eberhard, M.L., Njenga, M.N., DaSilva, A.J., Owino, D., Nace, E.K., Won, K.Y., Mwenda, J.M., 2001a. A survey for *Cyclospora* spp. in Kenyan primates, with some notes on its biology. J. Parasitol. 87, 1394–1397.

Eberhard, M.L., Njenga, M.N., DaSilva, A.J., Owino, D., Nace, E.K., Won, K.Y., Mwenda, J.M., 2001b. A survey for *Cyclospora* spp. in Kenyan primates, with some notes on its biology. J. Parasitol. 87, 1394–1397.

Eberhard, M.L., Owens, J.R., Bishop, H.S., de Almeida, M.E., da Silva, A.J., 2014. *Cyclospora* spp. in drills, Bioko Island, Equatorial Guinea. Emerg. Infect. Dis. 20, 510–511.

Elshazly, A.M., Elsheikha, H.M., Soltan, D.M., Mohammad, K.A., Morsy, T.A., 2007. Protozoal pollution of surface water sources in Dakahlia governorate, Egypt. J. Egypt. Soc. Parasitol. 37, 51–64.

Fryauff, D.J., Krippner, R., Prodjodipuro, P., Ewald, C., Kawengian, S., Pegelow, K., Yun, T., von Heydwolff-Wehnert, C., Oyofo, B., Gross, R., 1999. *Cyclospora cayetanensis* among expatriate and indigenous populations of West Java, Indonesia. Emerg. Infect. Dis. 5, 585–588.

Galván, A.L., Magnet, A., Izquierdo, F., Fenoy, S., Rueda, C., Fernández Vadillo, C., Henriques-Gil, N., del Aguila, C., 2013. Molecular characterization of human-pathogenic microsporidia and *Cyclospora cayetanensis* isolated from various water sources in Spain: a year-long longitudinal study. Appl. Environ. Microbiol. 79, 449–459.

García-López, H.L., Rodríguez-Tovar, L.E., Medina-De la Garza, C.E., 1996. Identification of *Cyclospora* in poultry. Emerg. Infect. Dis. 2, 356–357.

Ghozzi, K., Marangi, M., Papini, R., Lahmar, I., Challouf, R., Houas, N., Ben Dhiab, R., Normanno, G., Babba, H., Giangaspero, A., 2017. First report of Tunisian coastal water contamination by protozoan parasites using mollusk bivalves as biological indicators. Mar. Pollut. Bull. 117, 197–202.

Giangaspero, A., Gasser, R.B., 2019. Human cyclosporiasis. Lancet Infect. Dis. 19, e226–e236.

Giangaspero, A., Marangi, M., Koehler, A.V., Papini, R., Normanno, G., Lacasella, V., Lonigro, A., Gasser, R.B., 2015. Molecular detection of *Cyclospora* in water, soil, vegetables and humans in southern Italy signals a need for improved monitoring by health authorities. Int. J. Food Microbiol. 211, 95–100.

Graczyk, T.K., Ortega, Y.R., Conn, D.B., 1998. Recovery of waterborne oocysts of *Cyclospora cayetanensis* by Asian freshwater clams (*Corbicula fluminea*). Am. J. Trop. Med. Hyg. 59, 928–932.

Helenbrook, W.D., Wade, S.E., Shields, W.M., Stehman, S.V., Whipps, C.M., 2015. Gastrointestinal parasites of ecuadorian mantled howler monkeys (*Alouatta palliata aequatorialis*) based on fecal analysis. J. Parasitol. 101, 341–350.

Herwaldt, B.L., Ackers, M.L., 1997. An outbreak in 1996 of cyclosporiasis associated with imported raspberries. The Cyclospora Working Group. N. Engl. J. Med. 36, 1548–1556.

Jiang, Y., Yuan, Z., Zang, G., Li, D., Wang, Y., Zhang, Y., Liu, H., Cao, J., Shen, Y., 2018. *Cyclospora cayetanensis* infections among diarrheal outpatients in Shanghai: a retrospective case study. Front. Med. 12, 98–103.

Kaminsky, R.G., Lagos, J., Raudales Santos, G., Urrutia, S., 2016. Marked seasonality of *Cyclospora cayetanensis* infections: ten-year observation of hospital cases, Honduras. BMC Infect. Dis. 16, 66.

Karaman, Ü., Kolören, Z., Seferoğlu, O., Ayaz, E., Demirel, E., 2017. Presence of parasites in environmental waters in Samsun and its districts, Turkiye. Parazitol. Derg. 41, 19–21.

Khalifa, R.M., Ahmad, A.K., Abdel-Hafeez, E.H., Mosllem, F.A., 2014. Present status of protozoan pathogens causing water-borne disease in northern part of El-Minia governorate, Egypt. J. Egypt. Soc. Parasitol. 44, 559–566.

Kimura, K., Rai, S.K., Rai, G., Insisiengmay, S., Kawabata, M., Karanis, P., Uga, S., 2005. Study on *Cyclospora cayetanensis* associated with diarrheal disease in Nepal and Loa PDR. Southeast Asian J. Trop. Med. Public Health 36, 1371–1376.

Kitajima, M., Haramoto, E., Iker, B.C., Gerba, C.P., 2014. Occurrence of *Cryptosporidium*, *Giardia*, and *Cyclospora* in influent and effluent water at wastewater treatment plants in Arizona. Sci. Total Environ. 484, 129–136.

Kłudkowska, M., Pielok, Ł., Frąckowiak, K., Paul, M., 2017. Intestinal coccidian parasites as an underestimated cause of travellers' diarrhoea in Polish immunocompetent patients. Acta Parasitol. 62, 630–638.

Kwakye-Nuako, G., Borketey, P., Mensah-Attipoe, I., Asmah, R., Ayeh-Kumi, P., 2007. Sachet drinking water in Accra: the potential threats of transmission of enteric pathogenic protozoan organisms. Ghana Med. J. 41, 62–67.

Lee, H.Y., Stephen, A., Sushela, D., Mala, M., 2008. Detection of protozoan and bacterial pathogens of public health importance in faeces of *Corvus* spp. (large-billed crow). Trop. Biomed. 25, 134–139.

Legesse, M., Erko, B., 2004. Zoonotic intestinal parasites in *Papio anubis* (baboon) and *Cercopithecus aethiops* (vervet) from four localities in Ethiopia. Acta Trop. 90, 231–236.

Li, G., Xiao, S., Zhou, R., Li, W., Wadeh, H., 2007. Molecular characterization of *Cyclospora*-like organism from dairy cattle. Parasitol. Res. 100, 955–961.

Li, W., Kiulia, N.M., Mwenda, J.M., Nyachieo, A., Taylor, M.B., Zhang, X., Xiao, L., 2011. *Cyclospora papionis*, *Cryptosporidium hominis*, and human-pathogenic *Enterocytozoon bieneusi* in captive baboons in Kenya. J. Clin. Microbiol. 49, 4326–4329.

Li, N., Ye, J., Arrowood, M.J., Ma, J., Wang, L., Xu, H., Feng, Y., Xiao, L., 2015. Identification and morphologic and molecular characterization of *Cyclospora macacae* n. sp. from rhesus monkeys in China. Parasitol. Res. 114, 1811–1816.

Li, J., Dong, H., Wang, R., Yu, F., Wu, Y., Chang, Y., Wang, C., Qi, M., Zhang, L., 2017. An investigation of parasitic infections and review of molecular characterization of the intestinal protozoa in nonhuman primates in China from 2009 to 2015. Int. J. Parasitol. Parasites Wildl. 6, 8–15.

Li, J., Wang, R., Chen, Y., Xiao, L., Zhang, L., 2020. *Cyclospora cayetanensis* infection in humans: biological characteristics, clinical features, epidemiology, detection method, and treatment. Parasitology 147, 160–170.

Mansfield, L.S., Gajadhar, A.A., 2004. *Cyclospora cayetanensis*, a food- and waterborne coccidian parasite. Vet. Parasitol. 126, 73–90.

Marangi, M., Koehler, A.V., Zanzani, S.A., Manfredi, M.T., Brianti, E., Giangaspero, A., Gasser, R.B., 2015. Detection of *Cyclospora* in captive chimpanzees and macaques by a quantitative PCR-based mutation scanning approach. Parasit. Vectors 8, 274.

Mossallam, S.F., 2010. Detection of some intestinal protozoa in commercial fresh juices. J. Egypt. Soc. Parasitol. 40, 135–149.

Orozco-Mosqueda, G.E., Martínez-Loya, O.A., Ortega, Y.R., 2014. *Cyclospora cayetanensis* in a pediatric hospital in Morelia, México. Am. J. Trop. Med. Hyg. 91, 537–540.

Ortega, Y.R., Sanchez, R., 2010. Update on *Cyclospora cayetanensis*, a food-borne and water-borne parasite. Clin. Microbiol. Rev. 23, 218–234.

Ortega, Y.R., Roxas, C.R., Gilman, R.H., Miller, N.J., Cabrera, L., Taquiri, C., Sterling, C.R., 1997. Isolation of *Cryptosporidium parvum* and *Cyclospora cayetanensis* from vegetables collected in markets of an endemic region in Peru. Am. J. Trop. Med. Hyg. 57, 683–686.

Ozdamar, M., Hakko, E., Turkoglu, S., 2010. High occurrence of cyclosporiasis in Istanbul, Turkey, during a dry and warm summer. Parasit. Vectors 3, 39.

Pandey, P., Bodhidatta, L., Lewis, M., Murphy, H., Shlim, D.R., Cave, W., Rajah, R., Springer, M., Batchelor, T., Sornsakrin, S., Mason, C.J., 2011. Travelers' diarrhea in Nepal: an update on the pathogens and antibiotic resistance. J. Travel. Med. 18, 102–108.

Resendiz-Nava, C.N., Orozco-Mosqueda, G.E., Mercado-Silva, E.M., Flores-Robles, S., Silva-Rojas, H.V., Nava, G.M., 2020. A molecular tool for rapid detection and traceability of *Cyclospora cayetanensis* in fresh berries and berry farm soils. Foods 9, 261.

Robertson, L.J., Gjerde, B., Campbell, A.T., 2000. Isolation of *Cyclospora* oocysts from fruits and vegetables using lectin-coated paramagnetic beads. J. Food Prot. 63, 1410–1414.

Rose, J.B., Slifko, T.R., 1999. *Giardia*, *Cryptosporidium*, and *Cyclospora* and their impact on foods: a review. J. Food Prot. 62, 1059–1070.

Sherchand, J.B., Cross, J.H., 2001. Emerging pathogen *Cyclospora cayetanensis* infection in Nepal. Southeast Asian J. Trop. Med. Public Health 32, 143–150.

Shields, J.M., Olson, B.H., 2003. *Cyclospora cayetanensis*: a review of an emerging parasitic coccidian. Int. J. Parasitol. 33, 371–391.

Shields, J.M., Lee, M.M., Murphy, H.R., 2012. Use of a common laboratory glassware detergent improves recovery of *Cryptosporidium parvum* and *Cyclospora cayetanensis* from lettuce, herbs and raspberries. Int. J. Food Microbiol. 153, 123–128.

Sim, S., Won, J., Kim, J.W., Kim, K., Park, W.Y., Yu, J.R., 2017. Simultaneous molecular detection of *Cryptosporidium* and *Cyclospora* from raw vegetables in Korea. Korean J. Parasitol. 55, 137–142.

Smith, H.V., Paton, C.A., Girdwood, R.W., Mtambo, M.M., 1996. *Cyclospora* in non-human primates in Gombe, Tanzania. Vet. Rec. 138, 528.

Sturbaum, G.D., Ortega, Y.R., Gilman, R.H., Sterling, C.R., Cabrera, L., Klein, D.A., 1998. Detection of *Cyclospora cayetanensis* in wastewater. Appl. Environ. Microbiol. 64, 2284–2286.

Tefera, T., Biruksew, A., Mekonnen, Z., Eshetu, T., 2014. Parasitic contamination of fruits and vegetables collected from selected local markets of Jimma town, Southwest Ethiopia. Int. Sch. Res. Notices 2014, 382715.

Temesgen, T.T., Tysnes, K.R., Robertson, L.J., 2019. A new protocol for molecular detection of *Cyclospora cayetanensis* as contaminants of berry fruits. Front. Microbiol. 10, 1939.

Tram, N.T., Hoang, L.M., Cam, P.D., Chung, P.T., Fyfe, M.W., Isaac-Renton, J.L., Ong, C.S.L., 2008. *Cyclospora* spp. in herbs and water samples collected from markets and farms in Hanoi, Vietnam. Trop. Med. Int. Health 13, 1415–1420.

Vuong, T.A., Nguyen, T.T., Klank, L.T., Phung, D.C., Dalsgaard, A., 2007. Faecal and protozoan parasite contamination of water spinach (*Ipomoea aquatica*) cultivated in urban wastewater in Phnom Penh, Cambodia. Trop. Med. Int. Health. 12, 73–81.

Xiao, S.M., Li, G.Q., Zhou, R.Q., Li, W.H., Yang, J.W., 2007. Combined PCR-oligonucleotide ligation assay for detection of dairy cattle-derived *Cyclospora* sp. Vet. Parasitol. 149, 185–190.

Yai, L.E., Bauab, A.R., Hirschfeld, M.P., de Oliveira, M.L., Damaceno, J.T., 1997. The first two cases of *Cyclospora* in dogs, São Paulo, Brazil. Rev. Inst. Med. Trop. Sao Paulo 39, 177–179.

Yamada, M., Hatama, S., Ishikawa, Y., Kadota, K., 2014. Intranuclear coccidiosis caused by *Cyclospora* spp. in calves. J. Vet. Diagn. Investig. 26, 678–682.

Ye, J., Xiao, L., Li, J., Huang, W., Amer, S.E., Guo, Y., Roellig, D., Feng, Y., 2014. Occurrence of human-pathogenic *Enterocytozoon bieneusi*, *Giardia duodenalis* and *Cryptosporidium* genotypes in laboratory macaques in Guangxi, China. Parasitol. Int. 63, 132–137.

Zhao, G.H., Cong, M.M., Bian, Q.Q., Cheng, W.Y., Wang, R.J., Qi, M., Zhang, L.X., Lin, Q., Zhu, X.Q., 2013. Molecular characterization of *Cyclospora*-like organisms from golden snub-nosed monkeys in Qinling Mountain in Shaanxi province, northwestern China. PLoS One 8, e58216.

Zhou, Y., Lv, B., Wang, Q., Wang, R., Jian, F., Zhang, L., Ning, C., Fu, K., Wang, Y., Qi, M., Yao, H., Zhao, J., Zhang, X., Sun, Y., Shi, K., Arrowood, M.J., Xiao, L., 2011. Prevalence and molecular characterization of *Cyclospora cayetanensis*, Henan, China. Emerg. Infect. Dis. 17, 1887–1890.

CHAPTER 6

Detection methods

Contents

6.1 Introduction

Cyclospora cayetanensis is an important obligate intracellular protozoa widely distributed throughout the world (Soave, 1996; Connor et al., 1999), and this parasite was recognized as an emerging water- and foodborne coccidian pathogen of enteric diseases in endemic regions and many developed countries since mid-1990s (Herwaldt, 2000; Mansfield and Gajadhar, 2004). Human cyclosporiasis, caused by *C. cayetanensis*, can occur in both immunocompetent and immunocompromised (e.g., HIV-positive) residents and travelers, and even severe forms can occur in these people (see detail in Chapter 3). Remarkably, the water- and foodborne outbreaks and sporadic cases of cyclosporiasis were reported every year, especially during spring and summer months. Although *Cyclospora* infection is usually not fatal in humans, protracted diarrhea often leads to severe dehydration in infected patients, particularly in infants who are at greatest risk of severe dehydration and death. Furthermore, coinfections with some other opportunistic pathogens (e.g., *Cryptosporidium*) would make the infection worse (Giangaspero and Gasser, 2019).

Cyclospora and Cyclosporiasis
https://doi.org/10.1016/B978-0-12-821616-3.00010-2
135

Precise and accurate diagnose of diseases is key to cure patients and to block transmission of pathogens. Gastrointestinal symptoms are the main clinical features of cyclosporiasis, with diarrhea as the typical presentation (see detail in Chapter 3). However, diarrhea is suggestive but not indicative to specially diagnose cyclosporiasis for clinicians, since diarrhea may not be the presenting or predominant symptom for patients with *Cyclospora* infection (Soave, 1996). On the other hand, definitive diagnosis of cyclosporiasis can be obtained relying on laboratory detection of *Cyclospora* or its DNA in clinical test materials (e.g., feces, intestinal fluid and small bowel biopsy specimens) (Eberhard et al., 1997). In this chapter, the currently available methods for detecting and identifying infection of *Cyclospora* are briefly introduced, including traditional recognized microscopic procedures and novel modern testing technologies (e.g., flow cytometry, molecular methods).

6.2 Microscopy

Microscopic detection of the oocysts in fecal samples has been identified as the "gold standard" procedure for antemortem definitive diagnosis of a variety of protozoan infections, including *Cyclospora*. *Cyclospora* oocysts can be detected in clinical stool samples by using direct wet smears. In fresh unpreserved fecal samples, light microscopy showed *C. cayetanensis* as spherical, nonrefractile, hyaline, unsporulated oocysts with the diameter in the range from 8 to 10 μm, containing a 6–7-μm greenish morula and consisting of a hollow cluster of refractile, membrane-bound globules (Long et al., 1991; Brennan et al., 1996). However, clinically, *Cyclospora* infection is easily overlooked or confused with other common enteric protozoa (e.g. *Cryptosporidium parvum*), since the freshly passed oocysts without sporulation are relatively nondescript. Therefore, sporulation assay should be performed to confirm *Cyclospora* infection. Generally, fresh unfixed oocysts were placed in 2.5% potassium dichromate at room temperature (23–30°C), and oocysts will sporulate usually from 5 to 15 days (Eberhard et al., 1997). Two sporocysts are evident in one completely sporulated oocyst, and each sporocyst contains two sporozoites. Differential interference contrast (DIC) microscopy is recommended when examining sporulated oocysts in wet-mount preparations, since the sporozoites within each sporocyst are not accurately visualized by routine light microscopy (Chiodini, 1994; Eberhard et al., 1997).

Interestingly, marked autofluorescence is exhibited in the *Cyclospora* oocyst wall, making it easily identifiable by using epifluorescence microscopy

(Eberhard et al., 1997; Ortega and Sanchez, 2010). *Cyclospora* oocysts aut-ofluoresce white-blue when using a 330–380-nm excitation filter, while fluorescent green was seen with an excitation filter of 450–490 nm (Ortega and Sanchez, 2010). This marked autofluorescence characteristic is distinct with other common enteric protozoan parasites, e.g., no diagnostic value of weak autofluorescence for *Cryptosporidium* and the presence of autofluorescence in the interior of *Cysisospora* (Berlin et al., 1996; Eberhard et al., 1997). Additionally, adding a drop of D'Antoni's iodine would aid in microscopic examination by reducing the nonspecific background fluorescence (Berlin et al., 1996; Eberhard et al., 1997). Comparison study showed the sensitivity and specificity of epifluorescence microscopy equaled or exceeded bright-field examination (Eberhard et al., 1997). However, the time and storage conditions of the stool would influence the intensity of oocyst fluorescence, and the epifluorescent capability is also challenged in some laboratories (Eberhard et al., 1997; Ortega and Sanchez, 2010).

Notably, considering the fact of intermittent shedding and/or small numbers of oocysts in fecal samples of patients (Eberhard et al., 1997; Herwaldt, 2000; Ortega and Sanchez, 2010), multiple (up to three) fecal samples collected from the same patient at 2- or 3-day intervals and a concentration procedure (e.g., formalin-ether sedimentation, flotation using sucrose solution) before fecal examination are recommended to enhance the chance of detecting *Cyclospora* infection (Eberhard et al., 1997; Ortega and Sanchez, 2010). In addition, as an important foodborne and waterborne parasite, *C. cayetanensis* oocysts were found in environmental samples (e.g., water) and food (e.g., fruits, salad, berries, juice, vegetable). However, infections in these samples are more difficult to examine than fecal samples (Herwaldt, 2000). Suitable recovery procedures should be conducted before detection and combination with molecular technologies (see Section 6.4) would substantially improve the sensitivity (Herwaldt, 2000; Shields et al., 2012).

6.3 Flow cytometry

Based on the autofluorescence characteristic of *Cyclospora* oocysts, a detection procedure for human fecal samples by using flow cytometry was developed (Dixon et al., 2005). *Cyclospora* oocysts in SAF fixed human fecal samples were concentrated by using a sucrose gradient flotation procedure and analyzed with a FACScan equipped with an argon-ion laser operating at 488 nm and CellQuest software. *Cyclospora* oocysts were identified and clearly separated according to their autofluorescence, size, and complexity. Close correlation in terms of the presence or absence of oocysts was found between the flow cytometry and microscopy, and the sensitivity of flow cytometry appeared to be higher than microscopy. Furthermore, the sample preparation time for flow cytometry was similar to or slightly longer than that for microscopy, but the actual analysis time is much shorter. More importantly, as a largely automated method, it could omit the influence by an analyst's levels of fatigue and expertise for traditional microscopic technique. A comparative study conducted in fecal samples of pediatrics patients showed consistent results for symptomatic and asymptomatic patients and no significant differences in oocysts counts between flow cytometry and quantitative real-time PCR (Hussein et al., 2007). In addition to precise detection for *Cyclospora* oocysts, abilities of enumeration and large-scale sorting enabled flow cytometry to be a useful approach to screen *Cyclospora* oocysts in large numbers of fecal specimens (Dixon et al., 2005).

6.4 Staining methods

Several staining techniques have been developed to detect protozoan parasites on wet or dry mounts, including modified Ziehl-Neelsen (acid-fast), Kinyoun, lactophenol cotton blue, safranin, auramine, rhodamine, carbol fuchsin, Giemsa, and trichrome (Fletcher et al., 2012; Giangaspero and Gasser, 2019; Li et al., 2020a). The acid-fast staining has been identified as the standard method for detecting coccidian oocysts, e.g., *Cryptosporidium* and *Cystoisospora*, since there are acid-fast lipids in these parasites (Eberhard et al., 1997; Garcia et al., 2017; Li et al., 2020b). Similarly, due to this common property containing in *Cyclospora* oocysts, modified acid-fast staining can be used to identify this organism. However, marked variability is exhibited by *Cyclospora* oocysts in acid-fast staining (Eberhard et al., 1997), from no staining (so-called ghosts) or colorless to pink or deep purple (Visvesvara et al., 1997). More seriously, the structure of oocyst wall is variable in acid-fast stains, acquiring wrinkled or crinkled appearance, or collapsing or distorted on one or more sides (Eberhard et al., 1997; Mota et al., 2000). These problems would lead to possible misidentification of *Cyclospora* oocysts, indicating that the detection of this parasite in clinical samples using acid-fast staining alone is unreliable. Using DIC microscopy will be greatly helpful in the recognition of unstained oocysts (Eberhard et al., 1997; Mota et al., 2000). To improve the detection and visualization of *Cyclospora* oocysts in clinical samples, minor variations have been performed in modified acid-fast staining procedures, such as using 1%–3% H_2SO_4 as a decolorizer without alcohol, adding dimethyl sulfoxide (DMSO) to the phenol-basic fuchsine, and the incorporation of acetic acid with malachite green acting as a combined decolorizer-counterstain (Garcia et al., 2017; Almeria et al., 2019).

In 1997, a modified safranin technique was developed by Visvesvara et al.. In this procedure, the fecal smears were heated in a microwave oven at full power (650W) prior to staining, and almost all oocysts (98%) were uniformly stained with brilliant reddish orange. The sensitivity and specificity of this method was comparable with Ziehl-Neelsen acid-fast staining procedure (Visvesvara et al., 1997; Almeria et al., 2019). A similar heating procedure developed used a water bath at 85°C for 5 min instead of a microwave oven, and all oocysts in the smear being stained a bright red-orange without ghost oocysts (Maratim et al., 2002). Previous studies also showed that *Cyclospora* oocysts could not be effectively stained with Giemsa, trichrome, and Gram-chromotrope staining (Visvesvara et al., 1997; Mota et al., 2000; Ortega and Sanchez, 2010).

6.5 Molecular methods

6.5.1 Conventional PCR

In last decades, the small subunit ribosomal RNA (SSU rRNA, 18S rRNA) gene of *Cyclospora* was commonly used for the establishment of molecular detection protocols. In 1996, a nested PCR-based assay targeting hypervariable regions of 18S rRNA gene sequence of *Cyclospora* was first developed, with the target length of 308 bp (Relman et al., 1996). The sensitivity of this method was as few as ~10–50 cesium chloride gradient-purified oocysts, and no cross reactivity was found with DNA samples of some common pathogens, e.g., *Babesia microti*, *Neospora*, *C. parvum*, *Toxoplasma gondii*, and *Bordetella* (Relman et al., 1996). The sensitivity of this molecular technology was 40 or fewer oocysts per 100 g of raspberries or basil, but was ~1000 per 100 g in mesclun lettuce (Steele et al., 2003). This PCR assay also greatly improved diagnostic yield of *C. cayetanensis* cases in an outbreak of cyclosporiasis in Lima, Peru (Mundaca et al., 2008). However, this technology could not discriminate *Cyclospora* from *Eimeria* spp. (e.g., *Eimeria bovis*, *Eimeria nieschulzi*, and *Eimeria vermiformis*) (Relman et al., 1996) and primate *Cyclospora* spp. (Mansfield and Gajadhar, 2004). Low sensitivity (62%) was also found using this method in the detection of clinical stool samples (Eberhard et al., 1997). Another nested-PCR based on a segment of the

18S rRNA gene, with a slight modification to the protocol described by Relman et al. (1996), was also developed, generating a 294-bp amplicon in the presence of the *C. cayetanensis* template (Orlandi and Lampel, 2000). Positive amplification using this nested PCR was obtained with samples containing 0.3–10 oocysts per gram of fresh raspberries, corresponding to the detection limit of 30 oocysts in a 100 g fruit sample. Furthermore, the primers designed in this study could be used in multiplex PCR analysis with other two common protozoan parasites, *C. parvum* and *Encephalitozoon intestinalis*. Recently, Resendiz-Nava et al. (2020) generated a nested PCR using a combination of two pairs of previous primers (CYCF1E and CYCR2B, CC719 and CRP999) amplifying a segment of the 18S rRNA gene for *C. cayetanensis* (Relman et al., 1996; Orlandi et al., 2003), with the detection limit as few as 1 oocyst per gram of sample. This method could be used for rapid detection and traceability of *C. cayetanensis* in berries and berry farm soils. Unfortunately, the cross reactivity with *Eimeria* spp. was not evaluated for both nested PCR protocols.

Other than the 18S rRNA gene, the 70-kDa heat shock protein (HSP70) gene was also selected as the target to develop nested PCR. Sulaiman et al. (2013) established a two-step nested PCR protocol based on the HSP70 gene, with a final amplicon of 1276 bp. This assay could successfully detect 16 *C. cayetanensis* isolates from Nepal, Mexico, and Peru, providing another useful genetic tool for the rapid detection of *C. cayetanensis*. However, the specificity and clinical efficacy of this method should be investigated in the future.

Additionally, a single-round PCR protocol was also developed to reliably detect *C. cayetanensis* oocysts in water and basil wash sediment with high sensitivity and specificity (Lalonde and Gajadhar, 2008). This PCR assay used a pair of diagnostic primers (CCITS2-F and CCITS2-R) designed to anneal at unique signature sequence location in the ITS-2 region of *C. cayetanensis* to reliably detect a single oocyst, and did not yield amplicons for DNA templates from *E. vermiformis*, *Eimeria ahsata*, *Eimeria zvernii*, *Eimeria falciformis*, *Eimeria tenella*, *Sarcocystis cruzi*, *C. parvum*, *T. gondii*, *Giardia lamblia*, *Escherichia coli*, *Trichinella spiralis*, *Saccharomyces cerevisiae*, or ovine fecal DNA.

6.5.2 PCR-RFLP

To resolve the problem of indistinguishability between *Cyclospora* spp. and *Eimeria* spp. for the nested PCR developed by Relman et al. (1996), a PCR-restriction fragment length polymorphism (PCR-RFLP) method was developed using a restriction enzyme *Mnl*I to digest the amplicons of this nested PCR (Jinneman et al., 1996). This method could differentiate *Cyclospora* spp. from *Eimeria* spp. and is commonly used to detect *Cyclospora* infection in fecal samples, foodstuffs, leafy greens, and environmental waters. However, this nested PCR-RFLP protocol could not distinguish four *Cyclospora* species, due to no sequence differences in *Mnl*I sites among these organisms (Shields and Olson, 2003). In 2003, Shields and Olson reported another PCR-RFLP by using the restriction enzyme *Alu*I and new PCR outer (YCAO1 and YCAR1) and inner primer sets (CYCAI2 and CYCAR1), which could accurately identify *C. cayetanensis* from *C. colobi* and *Cyclospora cercopitheci*, and detect as few as one oocyst seeded into an autoclaved pellet flocculated from 10 L of surface water.

6.5.3 PCR-OLA

The oligonucleotide-ligation assay (OLA) is an SNP assay and can specifically investigate difference in single base pair by detecting ligation between capture probe and reporter probe. A PCR-OLA was developed based on the 18S rRNA gene region, with a 5′-phosphorylated reporter probe and a 5′-biotin labeled capture probes (Jinneman et al., 1999). This technique correctly differentiated three *Cyclospora*, three *E. tenella*, and one *Eimeria mitis* strains, and could be used to rapidly confirm amplified products of nested PCR for *Cyclospora* or *Eimeria* spp. In 2007, an enzyme-linked immunosorbent assay (ELISA)-based OLA has been developed to detect dairy cattle-derived *Cyclospora* sp. (Xiao et al., 2007). It was able to detect more than 0.5 ng of purified amplicons and was more sensitive than the common way with gel electrophoresis in detecting clinical samples.

6.5.4 qPCR-MCA

Several single or multiplex real-time PCR or protocols have been described to detect *C. cayetanensis* only or simultaneously with some common human pathogens (Qvarnstrom et al., 2018; Li et al., 2020a, b). A real-time quantitative PCR (qPCR) assay with fluorescent melting curve analysis (MCA) was also developed to simultaneously identify a groups of coccidian oocysts (including *Cyclospora*, *Toxoplasma*, *Eimeria*, *Sarcocystis*, *Cystoisospora*, and *Cryptosporidium*) (Lalonde and Gajadhar, 2011). After qPCR amplification using universal coccidia primer cocktail, these protozoan species could be differentiated by unique melting curves based on their specific melting temperatures (Tms). This assay has been successfully used to detect protozoan oocysts in human fecal samples in Dominican Republic, and four protozoan parasites including *C. cayetanensis* were identified, suggesting that it will be reliable protozoan oocyst screening assay for use on clinical and environmental samples in public health, food safety, and veterinary programs (Lalonde et al., 2013). Aksoy et al. (2014) also reported a real-time PCR/HRM to detect the presence of *T. gondii* and *C. cayetanensis* in *Mytilus galloprovincialis* from Izmir Province coast, Turkey, and first reported *T. gondii* Type 1, and *C. cayetanensis* in this edible shellfish in Turkey.

6.5.5 Multiplex-touchdown PCR

A multiplex-touchdown PCR has been reported to simultaneously detect three major protozoan parasites causing travelers' diarrhea, namely *C. parvum*, *G. lamblia*, and *C. cayetanensis*, with the target genes of the *Cryptosporidium* oocyst wall protein, Glutamate dehydrogenase, and 18S rRNA, respectively (Shin et al., 2016). The limit of detection were $> 1 \times 10^3$ oocysts for *C. parvum*, $> 1 \times 10^4$ cysts for *G. lamblia*, and > 1 copy of the 18S rRNA gene for *C. cayetanensis*, and this assay could be used to simultaneously diagnose infections of these protozoans in stool samples of humans and animals.

6.6 Serological testing

Serological tests through detecting antigen and/or specific antibodies have been proved to be useful in sporadic cases and epidemiological studies (especially in outbreak investigations) (Ortega and Sanchez, 2010; Li et al., 2020a, b). However, due to lack of specific monoclonal antibodies against oocysts of *C. cayetanensis*, no commercial serological testing methods were available to specially determine *Cyclospora* infection on an individual patient level and oocysts in environmental samples and foods to the best of our knowledge (Quintero-Betancourt et al., 2002; Almeria et al., 2019; Giangaspero and Gasser, 2019; Li et al., 2020a, b). An immunofluorescent-antibody (IFA) microscopy has been used to investigate a serological immune response in patients infected with *C. cayetanensis* (Clarke and McIntyre, 1997). An ELISA method was developed to detect IgG and IgM in patients with *Cyclospora* oocysts from several regions in Anhui Province of China (Wang et al., 2002). The embraced antigen of this technique was oocysts of *C. cayetanensis* from artificially infected guinea pigs, and a positive sample was judged when it was 2.1 times as much as the negative. A Western blot assay has also been developed to identify acute- from convalescent-phase cyclosporiasis (Ortega and Sanchez, 2010). However, several serious limitations greatly restrict these serological assays. For example, a large number of oocysts are needed but suitable animal models and in vitro culture systems to propagate *Cyclospora* oocysts are lacking (Ortega and Sanchez, 2010; Li et al., 2020a, b). The reproducibility and validity of these methods are another constrain and should be performed by other scientists (Ortega and Sanchez, 2010).

6.7 Conclusion

Over the last decades, a great number of detection methods were developed to investigate *Cyclospora* oocysts in stools, vehicles (e.g., fresh produces, leafy greens), and environmental water and soil, and they greatly assisted laboratorians and investigators to accurately identify *Cyclospora* involved in several sporadic cases or outbreaks. However, clinically, there are still no standard or commercial protocols to detect *Cyclospora* infection due to defect in each available method. Generally, conventional microscopy with or without staining visually displays the presence of *Cyclospora* oocysts in samples but needs expertising microscopists and suitable concentration procedures, specifically for low number of oocysts, while modern molecular detection provides a specific and sensitive protocol for diagnosing *Cyclospora* in clinical or epidemiological settings but cannot determine viability and infectivity of *Cyclospora* oocysts. Therefore, combined application of molecular tools with microscopic methods would be a reasonable direction for constructing suitable detection systems for *C. cayetanensis* and other *Cyclospora* species. Recently, sequences of mitochondrial, apicoplast, and whole genomes were obtained and analyzed, providing useful information to develop novel molecular tools to detect *Cyclospora* infection in source tracking and case clusters. Furthermore, it is expected that breakthroughs made in animal models and in vitro culture systems will facilitate research and control on *C. cayetanensis*.

References

Aksoy, U., Marangi, M., Papini, R., Ozkoc, S., Bayram Delibas, S., Giangaspero, A., 2014. Detection of *Toxoplasma gondii* and *Cyclospora cayetanensis* in *Mytilus galloprovincialis* from Izmir Province coast (Turkey) by real time PCR/high-resolution melting analysis (HRM). Food Microbiol. 44, 128–135.
Almeria, S., Cinar, H.N., Dubey, J.P., 2019. *Cyclospora cayetanensis* and Cyclosporiasis: an update. Microorganisms 7 (9), 317.
Berlin, O.G., Conteas, C.N., Sowerby, T.M., 1996. Detection of *Isospora* in the stools of AIDS patients using a new rapid autofluorescence technique. AIDS 10 (4), 442–443.
Brennan, M.K., MacPherson, D.W., Palmer, J., Keystone, J.S., 1996. Cyclosporiasis: a new cause of diarrhea. CMAJ 155 (9), 1293–1296.
Chiodini, P.L., 1994. A 'new' parasite: human infection with *Cyclospora cayetanensis*. Trans. R. Soc. Trop. Med. Hyg. 88 (4), 369–371.

Clarke, S.C., McIntyre, M., 1997. An attempt to demonstrate a serological immune response in patients infected with *Cyclospora cayetanensis*. Br. J. Biomed. Sci. 54 (1), 73–74.

Connor, B.A., Reidy, J., Soave, R., 1999. Cyclosporiasis: clinical and histopathologic correlates. Clin. Infect. Dis. 28 (6), 1216–1222.

Dixon, B.R., Bussey, J.M., Parrington, L.J., Parenteau, M., 2005. Detection of *Cyclospora cayetanensis* oocysts in human fecal specimens by flow cytometry. J. Clin. Microbiol. 43 (5), 2375–2379.

Eberhard, M.L., Pieniazek, N.J., Arrowood, M.J., 1997. Laboratory diagnosis of Cyclospora infections. Arch. Pathol. Lab. Med. 121 (8), 792–797.

Fletcher, S.M., Stark, D., Harkness, J., Ellis, J., 2012. Enteric protozoa in the developed world: a public health perspective. Clin. Microbiol. Rev. 25 (3), 420–449.

Garcia, L.S., Arrowood, M., Kokoskin, E., Paltridge, G.P., Pillai, D.R., Procop, G.W., Ryan, N., Shimizu, R.Y., Visvesvara, G., 2017. Practical guidance for clinical microbiology laboratories: laboratory diagnosis of parasites from the gastrointestinal tract. Clin. Microbiol. Rev. 31 (4), e00025-17.

Giangaspero, A., Gasser, R.B., 2019. Human cyclosporiasis. Lancet Infect. Dis. 19 (7), e226–e236.

Herwaldt, B.L., 2000. *Cyclospora cayetanensis*: a review, focusing on the outbreaks of cyclosporiasis in the 1990s. Clin. Infect. Dis. 31 (4), 1040–1057.

Hussein, E.M., El-Moamly, A.A., Dawoud, H.A., Fahmy, H., El-Shal, H.E., Sabek, N.A., 2007. Real-time PCR and Flow cytometry in detection of *Cyclospora* oocysts in fecal samples of symptomatic and asymptomatic pediatrics patients. J. Egypt. Soc. Parasitol. 37 (1), 151–170.

Jinneman, K.C., Wetherington, J.H., Adams, A.M., Johnson, J.M., Tenge, B.J., Dang, N.L., Hill, W.E., 1996. Differentiation of *Cyclospora* sp. and *Eimeria* spp. by using the polymerase chain reaction amplification products and restriction fragment length polymorphisms. Food and Drug Administration Laboratory Information Bulletin. LIB no. 4044 [Online] http://vm.cfsan.fda.gov/mow/kjcs19c.html.

Jinneman, K.C., Wetherington, J.H., Hill, W.E., Omiescinski, C.J., Adams, A.M., Johnson, J.M., Tenge, B.J., Dang, N.L., Wekell, M.M., 1999. An oligonucleotide-ligation assay for the differentiation between *Cyclospora* and *Eimeria* spp. polymerase chain reaction amplification products. J. Food Prot. 62 (6), 682–685.

Lalonde, L.F., Gajadhar, A.A., 2008. Highly sensitive and specific PCR assay for reliable detection of *Cyclospora cayetanensis* oocysts. Appl. Environ. Microbiol. 74 (14), 4354–4358.

Lalonde, L.F., Gajadhar, A.A., 2011. Detection and differentiation of coccidian oocysts by real-time PCR and melting curve analysis. J. Parasitol. 97 (4), 725–730.

Lalonde, L.F., Reyes, J., Gajadhar, A.A., 2013. Application of a qPCR assay with melting curve analysis for detection and differentiation of protozoan oocysts in human fecal samples from Dominican Republic. Am. J. Trop. Med. Hyg. 89 (5), 892–898.

Li, J., Wang, R., Chen, Y., Xiao, L., Zhang, L., 2020a. *Cyclospora cayetanensis* infection in humans: biological characteristics, clinical features, epidemiology, detection method and treatment. Parasitology 147 (2), 160–170.

Li, J., Cui, Z., Qi, M., Zhang, L., 2020b. Advances in Cyclosporiasis diagnosis and therapeutic intervention. Front. Cell. Infect. Microbiol. 10, 43.

Long, E.G., White, E.H., Carmichael, W.W., Quinlisk, P.M., Raja, R., Swisher, B.L., Daugharty, H., Cohen, M.T., 1991. Morphologic and staining characteristics of a cyanobacterium-like organism associated with diarrhea. J Infect Dis 164 (1), 199–202.

Mansfield, L.S., Gajadhar, A.A., 2004. *Cyclospora cayetanensis*, a food- and waterborne coccidian parasite. Vet. Parasitol. 126 (1–2), 73–90.

Maratim, A.C., Kamar, K.K., Ngindu, A., Akoru, C.N., Diero, L., Sidle, J., 2002. Safranin staining of *Cyclospora cayetanensis* oocysts not requiring microwave heating. Br. J. Biomed. Sci. 59 (2), 114–115.

Mota, P., Rauch, C.A., Edberg, S.C., 2000. Microsporidia and *Cyclospora*: epidemiology and assessment of risk from the environment. Crit. Rev. Microbiol. 26 (2), 69–90.

Mundaca, C.C., Torres-Slimming, P.A., Araujo-Castillo, R.V., Morán, M., Bacon, D.J., Ortega, Y., Gilman, R.H., Blazes, D.L., 2008. Use of PCR to improve diagnostic yield in an outbreak of cyclosporiasis in Lima, Peru. Trans. R. Soc. Trop. Med. Hyg. 102 (7), 712–717.

Orlandi, P.A., Lampel, K.A., 2000. Extraction-free, filter-based template preparation for rapid and sensitive PCR detection of pathogenic parasitic protozoa. J. Clin. Microbiol. 38 (6), 2271–2277.

Orlandi, P.A., Carter, L., Brinker, A.M., da Silva, A.J., Chu, D.M., Lampel, K.A., Monday, S.R., 2003. Targeting single-nucleotide polymorphisms in the 18S rRNA gene to differentiate *Cyclospora* species from *Eimeria* species by multiplex PCR. Appl. Environ. Microbiol. 69 (8), 4806–4813.

Ortega, Y.R., Sanchez, R., 2010. Update on *Cyclospora cayetanensis*, a food-borne and water-borne parasite. Clin. Microbiol. Rev. 23 (1), 218–234.

Quintero-Betancourt, W., Peele, E.R., Rose, J.B., 2002. Cryptosporidium parvum and *Cyclospora cayetanensis*: a review of laboratory methods for detection of these waterborne parasites. J. Microbiol. Methods 49 (3), 209–224.

Qvarnstrom, Y., Benedict, T., Marcet, P.L., Wiegand, R.E., Herwaldt, B.L., da Silva, A.J., 2018. Molecular detection of *Cyclospora cayetanensis* in human stool specimens using UNEX-based DNA extraction and real-time PCR. Parasitology 145 (7), 865–870.

Relman, D.A., Schmidt, T.M., Gajadhar, A., Sogin, M., Cross, J., Yoder, K., Sethabutr, O., Echeverria, P., 1996. Molecular phylogenetic analysis of *Cyclospora*, the human intestinal pathogen, suggests that it is closely related to *Eimeria* species. J Infect Dis 173 (2), 440–445.

Resendiz-Nava, C.N., Orozco-Mosqueda, G.E., Mercado-Silva, E.M., Flores-Robles, S., Silva-Rojas, H.V., Nava, G.M., 2020. A molecular tool for rapid detection and traceability of *Cyclospora cayetanensis* in fresh berries and berry farm soils. Foods 9 (3), 261.

Shields, J.M., Olson, B.H., 2003. PCR-restriction fragment length polymorphism method for detection of *Cyclospora cayetanensis* in environmental waters without microscopic confirmation. Appl. Environ. Microbiol. 69 (8), 4662–4669.

Shields, J.M., Lee, M.M., Murphy, H.R., 2012. Use of a common laboratory glassware detergent improves recovery of *Cryptosporidium parvum* and *Cyclospora cayetanensis* from lettuce, herbs and raspberries. Int. J. Food Microbiol. 153 (1–2), 123–128.

Shin, J.H., Lee, S.E., Kim, T.S., Ma, D.W., Chai, J.Y., Shin, E.H., 2016. Multiplex-touchdown PCR to simultaneously detect *Cryptosporidium parvum, Giardia lamblia*, and *Cyclospora cayetanensis*, the major causes of traveler's diarrhea. Korean J. Parasitol. 54 (5), 631–636.

Soave, R., 1996. Cyclospora: an overview. Clin. Infect. Dis. 23 (3), 429–437.

Steele, M., Unger, S., Odumeru, J., 2003. Sensitivity of PCR detection of *Cyclospora cayetanensis* in raspberries, basil, and mesclun lettuce. J. Microbiol. Methods 54 (2), 277–280.

Sulaiman, I.M., Torres, P., Simpson, S., Kerdahi, K., Ortega, Y., 2013. Sequence characterization of heat shock protein gene of *Cyclospora cayetanensis* isolates from Nepal, Mexico, and Peru. J. Parasitol. 99 (2), 379–382.

Visvesvara, G.S., Moura, H., Kovacs-Nace, E., Wallace, S., Eberhard, M.L., 1997. Uniform staining of Cyclospora oocysts in fecal smears by a modified safranin technique with microwave heating. J. Clin. Microbiol. 35 (3), 730–733.

Wang, K.X., Li, C.P., Wang, J., Tian, Y., 2002. *Cyclospore cayetanensis* in Anhui, China. World J. Gastroenterol. 8 (6), 1144–1148.

Xiao, S.M., Li, G.Q., Zhou, R.Q., Li, W.H., Yang, J.W., 2007. Combined PCR-oligonucleotide ligation assay for detection of dairy cattle-derived *Cyclospora* sp. Vet. Parasitol. 149 (3–4), 185–190.

CHAPTER 7

Treatment and prevention

Contents

7.1 Introduction

Significant advances have been achieved in our knowledge of the biology, pathogenesis, diagnosis, and control of cyclosporiasis during the past decades (Li et al., 2020a, b). These help us to better understand this foodborne parasite and to explore effective anti-*Cyclospora* medicines and/ or prevention and control measures. Although no vaccine is available for cyclosporiasis, early detection and treatment can yield a favorable clinical outcome. For example, treatment with TMP-SMX has proven effective for cyclosporiasis. Ciprofloxacin, although less effective than TMP-SMX, can suitably be used in patients having sulfur drug intolerance. Nitazoxanide is an alternative drug that can be used in the cases of sulfur intolerance and ciprofloxacin resistance (Li et al., 2020a). Nevertheless, several factors affect the likelihood of infective oocysts of *Cyclospora cayetanensis* contaminating food due for human consumption, including the way in which the food is produced, harvested, transported, stored, prepared, and consumed. Being aware of these factors is an essential step in identifying critical control points during this chain, such that preventive measures to reduce the likelihood of contamination can be implemented (Ortega and Robertson, 2017). In this chapter, we have selected to survey and compile the available scientific literature regarding chemotherapy and prevention and control measures.

Cyclospora and Cyclosporiasis
https://doi.org/10.1016/B978-0-12-821616-3.00004-7
147

7.2 Therapy

Currently, no vaccine is available for cyclosporiasis (Giangaspero and Gasser, 2019), however early detection and treatment can yield a favorable clinical outcome. Expectant treatment and chemotherapeutic treatment are crucial in human cyclosporiasis, particularly in immune-deficient individuals. Although case fatality due to cyclosporiasis is rare in humans, long-lasting diarrhea sometimes results in dehydration or malnutrition, and occasionally may cause severe dehydration and death in infants (Behera et al., 2008; Bednarska et al., 2015).

Chemotherapy including treatment with 160 mg trimethoprim and 800 mg sulfamethoxazole (TMP-SMX, also known as co-trimoxazole) twice daily for 7 days can reportedly cure human cyclosporiasis (Hoge et al., 1995; Escobedo et al., 2009). TMP-SMX is considered as an effective drug, with many studies reporting low recurrence rates (Hoge et al., 1995; Madico et al., 1997; Goldberg and Bishara, 2012). It is also an effective chemotherapeutic treatment for *C. cayetanensis* infection in AIDS patients (Pape et al., 1994; Verdier et al., 2000) and those with biliary disease (Sifuentes-Osornio et al., 1995).

In some patients, TMP-SMX creates intolerance and allergy. In such cases, ciprofloxacin antibiotic with having less effectivity than TMP-SMX is a suitable treatment option for cyclosporiasis in human (Verdier et al., 2000). Nitazoxanide is another drug that can also be used in the cases of sulfonamide intolerance and ciprofloxacin resistance (Diaz et al., 2003; Cohen, 2005; Zimmer et al., 2007). Nitazoxanide has been used to treat mixed parasite infection with intestinal protozoa (including *C. cayetanensis*) and helminths (Diaz et al., 2003). The efficacy of nitazoxanide for cyclosporiasis was reported to range from 71% to 87%. The tolerance level of the drug was found to be very high with serious adverse effects (Table 7.1). Conversely, norfloxacin, metronidazole, tinidazole, and quinacrine have proven ineffective in some studies of human cyclosporiasis (Escobedo et al., 2009; Almeria et al., 2019). In a more recent study in mice, silver nanoparticles were effective against *Cyclospora* infection (Gaafar et al., 2019). This will draw attention to its potential for use as an alternative to the standard therapy in both immune-competent and immune-suppressed hosts.

In immunocompromised patients with HIV-related disease, immune reconstitution using HAART, which acts prophylactically, is the treatment of choice. HAART reduces viral load and may also reduce parasite load. Protease inhibitors used in HAART reduce *C. parvum* sporozoite host-cell

Table 7.1 Anti-*Cyclospora* oocyst drugs.

Drugs	Dosages	Applicable population (scope)	References
TMP-SMX	(160 mg trimethoprim, 800 mg sulphamethoxazole) twice daily for 7 days	AIDS patients and those of them with biliary disease; an effective treatment with a low recurrence rate	Hoge et al. (1995), Madico et al. (1997), and Goldberg and Bishara (2012)
Ciprofloxacin	500 mg twice daily for 7 days	Patients with intolerance to sulfonamide drugs	Verdier et al. (2000)
Nitazoxanide	100 mg (9.52 mg/kg bwt) twice daily for 3 days	Patients having sulfur intolerance or for whom treatment with sulfa or ciprofloxacin has failed	Cohen (2005) and Zimmer et al. (2007)
Silver nanoparticles (NPs)	10 μg/mice i.p. once daily for 7 days	Only in experimental mice; effectiveness against *Cyclospora* infection	Gaafar et al. (2019)
Magnesium oxide (MgO) nanoparticles (NPs)[a]	12.5 mg/mL for 3 days	Anti-*Cyclospora* effect on both unsporulated and sporulated oocysts in food and water disinfectant treatment	Hussein et al. (2018)

Note: TMP-SMX, trimethoprim-sulfamethoxazole (also known as co-trimoxazole).

[a] For disinfection of food and water potentially containing oocysts.

invasion and parasite development in vitro, and inhibition is enhanced in combination with paromomycin (Hommer et al., 2003). HAART, in combination with antiparasitic therapy, may enhance *Cyclospora* clearance. In non-HIV immunosuppressed patients with cyclosporiasis, reducing immunosuppression prior to specific chemotherapy is a useful option.

7.3 Prevention and control

C. cayetanensis is contracted via a fecal-oral transmission cycle, and direct person-to-person transmission seems unlikely because the excreted oocysts are not infectious and require more than 7 days outside the host to sporulate. In developed nations, *C. cayetanensis* infections can be common in people who travel to endemic areas of underdeveloped and developing countries and consume the contaminated food, especially fresh produce imported from those regions (Almeria et al., 2019).

   C. cayetanensis is mainly transmitted via fecal contamination of food, water, and soil (Almeria et al., 2019). Therefore, strategies to prevent foodborne and waterborne contamination should therefore target the reduction or prevention of human infections and strive for improved sanitation. Proper hygiene habits and food washing and sanitizing may reduce, but should not be expected to eliminate, the risk of acquiring infections. It has been demonstrated that these practices do not completely remove *Cyclospora* oocysts from contaminated produce (Robertson et al., 2000). Good agricultural practices would indeed contribute to reducing the burden of parasite contamination at the farm level. These practices would involve the use of properly treated irrigation water and the use of pathogen-free water for washing produce.

   Several practices have been tested for the inactivation or reduction of the number of viable parasites in foods and in water. Because of the lack of animal or in vitro infectivity models, oocyst sporulation has been used as an indicator of viability. Methods that rely on temperature and time of storage have been evaluated for killing parasites. For dairy substrates, storage at $-15°C$ for 24h did not inactivate *Cyclospora* oocysts. For basil or water, storage at $-20°C$ for 2 days, 50°C for 1h, and 37°C for up to 4 days did not prevent *Cyclospora* sporulation; however, extreme temperatures (70°C, $-70°C$, and 100°C) were effective in preventing oocysts from sporulating (Ortega et al., 2008). Temperatures frequently used for produce storage, e.g., 4–23°C, do not affect sporulation of *Cyclospora*. Microwave heating of *Cyclospora* oocysts can inactivate oocysts; however, more time is required to kill *Cyclospora* oocysts than to kill *Cryptosporidium* oocysts. Short exposures to a high temperature (96°C for 45 s) did not completely prevent the sporulation of *Cyclospora* (Ortega and Liao, 2006). Chemicals have been tested for the ability to interfere with the sporulation of *Cyclospora*. Gaseous chlorine dioxide at 4.1 mg/L does not affect the sporulation of *Cyclospora*; however, this treatment does inactivate *Cryptosporidium* and microsporidia (Ortega et al., 2008).

The practice of not consuming raw fresh produce, especially those supplied from endemic areas, can avert the problem of cyclosporiasis in humans. Regular boiling and filtering of water necessary for drinking, food preparation, and washing of fresh produce can also prevent the infection (Almeria et al., 2019). While usual sanitizers and disinfectants cannot destroy *C. cayetanensis* and coccidia in general, some exploratory methods for removing or inactivating *C. cayetanensis* oocysts in fresh fruits and raw vegetables have been investigated (El Zawawy et al., 2010; Butot et al., 2018; Hussein et al., 2018). In one study magnesium oxide nanoparticles were found to have a significant anti-*Cyclospora* effect on both unsporulated and sporulated oocysts, prompting speculation that it may be useful as a preventive agent in food and water disinfection treatment (Hussein et al., 2018).

Care should be taken to keep the fresh produce out of contamination at the field and packaging unit, and also from the farm workers to effectively prevent the *C. cayetanensis* infection in endemic areas. The practice of toilet use, hand washing after toilet use and before meal, and proper disposal and treatment of human excreta are also important for the prevention of cyclosporiasis. Any worker bearing the gastrointestinal diseases should not handle the vegetables or other produce. Other coccidiosis control measures can also be applied for the prevention and control of *C. cayetanensis* infections.

The lack of in vivo or in vitro methods to test viability has prompted researchers to use surrogate parasites, such as *Eimeria* and *Toxoplasma gondii*, to evaluate other treatments. Gamma irradiation (137Cs) of sporulated and unsporulated *T. gondii* oocysts was evaluated as a model system for the inactivation of *Cyclospora* oocysts (Dubey et al., 1998). *T. gondii* oocysts treated with 0.4 kGy irradiation could sporulate, excyst, and infect cells but did not cause infections in mice. It was recommended that 0.5 kGy irradiation could be used to kill coccidian oocysts on fruits and vegetables (Dubey et al., 1998). Inactivation of *Eimeria acervulina* oocysts was achieved by freezing, heating, and irradiation at 1 kGy and higher (Lee and Lee, 2001).

High hydrostatic pressure (550 MPa at 40°C for 2 min) and UV light (up to 261 mW/cm^2) treatments of produce contaminated with *E. acervulina* as a

Cyclospora surrogate were evaluated on experimentally inoculated basil and raspberries (Kniel et al., 2007). Both treatments yielded smaller number of animals infected with *E. acervulina* but did not completely inactivate the oocysts recovered from these food matrices. *Toxoplasma* oocysts (VEG strain) inoculated onto raspberries were rendered noninfectious to mice when a high-pressure processing treatment of 340 MPa for 60 s was applied (Lindsay et al., 2008).

7.4 Conclusion

TMP-SMX has been proven effective treatment drug for human cyclosporiasis, with ciprofloxacin and nitazoxanide being the two alternative drugs. Little is known about the treatment measures aimed to *Cyclospora* infection in animals. Magnesium oxide (MgO) nanoparticles, having anti-*Cyclospora* effect on both unsporulated and sporulated oocysts in food and water disinfectant treatment, will provide useful approach to prevent foodborne and waterborne contamination, thus reducing or preventing human infections. Nevertheless, basic measures to prevent *Cyclospora* infection are necessarily emphasized, involving health education, correct personal hygiene, adequate hand washing, changes in eating habits, drinking boiled or bottled water and not eating raw produce, proper sanitary infrastructure, and the treatment of human sewage.

References

Almeria, S., Cinar, H.N., Dubey, J.P., 2019. *Cyclospora cayetanensis* and cyclosporiasis: an update. Microorganisms 7, 317.

Bednarska, M., Bajer, A., Welc-Faleciak, R., Pawelas, A., 2015. *Cyclospora cayetanensis* infection in transplant traveller: a case report of outbreak. Parasit.Vectors 8, 411.

Behera, B., Mirdha, B.R., Makharia, G.K., Bhatnagar, S., Dattagupta, S., Samantaray, J.C., 2008. Parasites in patients with malabsorption syndrome: a clinical study in children and adults. Dig. Dis. Sci. 53, 672–679.

Butot, S., Cantergiani, F., Moser, M., Jean, J., Lima, A., Michot, L., et al., 2018. UV-C inactivation of foodborne bacterial and viral pathogens and surrogates on fresh and frozen-berries. Int. J. Food Microbiol. 275, 8–16.

Cohen, S.A., 2005. Use of nitazoxanide as a new therapeutic option for persistent diarrhea: a pediatric perspective. Curr. Med. Res. Opin. 21, 999–1004.

Diaz, E., Mondragon, J., Ramirez, E., Bernal, R., 2003. Epidemiology and control of intestinal parasites with nitazoxanide in children in Mexico. Am. J. Trop. Med. Hyg. 68, 384–385.

Dubey, J.P., Thayer, D.W., Speer, C.A., Shen, S.K., 1998. Effect of gamma irradiation on unsporulated and sporulated *Toxoplasma gondii* oocysts. Int. J. Parasitol. 28, 369–375.

El Zawawy, L.A., El-Said, D., Ali, S.M., Fathy, F.M., 2010. Disinfection efficacy of sodium dichlorois ocyanurate (NADCC) against common food-borne intestinal protozoa. J. Egypt. Soc. Parasitol. 40, 165–185.

Escobedo, A.A., Almirall, P., Alfonso, M., Cimerman, S., Rey, S., Terry, S.L., 2009. Treatment of intestinal protozoan infections in children. Arch. Dis. Child. 94, 478–482.

Gaafar, M.R., El-Zawawy, L.A., El-Temsahy, M.M., Shalaby, T.I., Hassan, A.Y., 2019. Silver nanoparticles as a therapeutic agent in experimental cyclosporiasis. Exp. Parasitol. 207, 107772.

Giangaspero, A., Gasser, R.B., 2019. Human cyclosporiasis. Lancet Infect. Dis. 19, e226–e236.

Goldberg, E., Bishara, J., 2012. Contemporary unconventional clinical use of co-trimoxazole. Clin. Microbiol. Infect. 18, 8–17.

Hoge, C.W., Shlim, D.R., Ghimire, M., Rabold, J.G., Pandey, P., Walch, A., et al., 1995. Placebo-controlled trial of co-trimoxazole for *Cyclospora* infections among travellers and foreign residents in Nepal. Lancet 345, 691–693.

Hommer, V., Eichholz, J., Petry, F., 2003. Effect of antiretroviral protease inhibitors alone, and in combination with paromomycin, on the excystation, invasion and in vitro development of *Cryptosporidium parvum*. J. Antimicrob. Chemother. 52, 359–364.

Hussein, E.M., Ahmed, S.A., Mokhtar, A.B., Elzagawy, S.M., Yahi, S.H., Hussein, A.M., et al., 2018. Antiprotozoal activity of magnesium oxide (MgO) nanoparticles against *Cyclospora cayetanensis* oocysts. Parasitol. Int. 67, 666–674.

Kniel, K.E., Shearer, A.E., Cascarino, J.L., Wilkins, G.C., Jenkins, M.C., 2007. High hydrostatic pressure and UV light treatment of produce contaminated with Eimeria acervulina as a *Cyclospora cayetanensis* surrogate. J. Food Prot. 70, 2837–2842.

Lee, M.B., Lee, E.H., 2001. Coccidial contamination of raspberries: mock contamination with Eimeria acervulina as a model for decontamination treatment studies. J. Food Prot. 64, 1854–1857.

Li, J., Cui, Z., Qi, M., Zhang, L., 2020a. Advances in cyclosporiasis diagnosis and therapeutic intervention. Front. Cell. Infect. Microbiol. 10, 43.

Li, J., Wang, R., Chen, Y., Xiao, L., Zhang, L., 2020b. *Cyclospora cayetanensis* infection in humans: biological characteristics, clinical features, epidemiology, detection method and treatment. Parasitology 147, 160–170.

Lindsay, D.S., Holliman, D., Flick, G.J., Goodwin, D.G., Mitchell, S.M., Dubey, J.P., 2008. Effects of high pressure processing on *Toxoplasma gondii* oocysts on raspberries. J. Parasitol. 94, 757–758.

Madico, G., McDonald, J., Gilman, R.H., Cabrera, L., Sterling, C.R., 1997. Epidemiology and treatment of *Cyclospora cayetanensis* infection in Peruvian children. Clin. Infect. Dis. 24, 977–981.

Ortega, Y.R., Liao, J., 2006. Microwave inactivation of *Cyclospora cayetanensis* sporulation and viability of *Cryptosporidium parvum* oocysts. J. Food Prot. 69, 1957–1960.

Ortega, Y.R., Robertson, L.J., 2017. *Cyclospora cayetanensis* as a foodborne pathogen. In: SpringerBriefs in Food, Health, and Nutrition. Gewerbestrasse 11, 6330 Cham, Switzerland.

Ortega, Y.R., Mann, A., Torres, M.P., Cama, V., 2008. Efficacy of gaseous chlorine dioxide as a sanitizer against *Cryptosporidium parvum*, *Cyclospora cayetanensis*, and *Encephalitozoon intestinalis* on produce. J. Food Prot. 71, 2410–2414.

Pape, J.W., Verdier, R.I., Boncy, M., Boncy, J., Johnson Jr., W.D., 1994. *Cyclospora* infection in adults infected with HIV-clinical manifestations, treatment, and prophylaxis. Ann. Intern. Med. 121, 654–657.

Robertson, L.J., Gjerde, B., Campbell, A.T., 2000. Isolation of *Cyclospora* oocysts from fruits and vegetables using lectin-coated paramagnetic beads. J. Food Prot. 63, 1410–1414.

Sifuentes-Osornio, J., Porras-Cortés, G., Bendall, R.P., Morales-Villarreal, F., Reyes-Terán, G., Ruiz-Palacios, G.M., 1995. *Cyclospora cayetanensis* infection in patients with and without AIDS: biliary disease as another clinical manifestation. Clin. Infect. Dis. 21, 1092–1097.

Verdier, R.I., Fitzgerald, D.W., Johnson Jr., W.D., Pape, J.W., 2000. Trimethoprim-sulfamethoxazole compared with ciprofloxacin for treatment and prophylaxis of *Isospora belli* and *Cyclospora cayetanensis* infection in HIV-infected patients. A randomized, controlled trial. Ann. Intern. Med. 132, 885–888.

Zimmer, S.M., Schuetz, A.N., Franco-Paredes, C., 2007. Efficacy of nitazoxanide for cyclosporiasis in patients with sulfa allergy. Clin. Infect. Dis. 44, 466–467.

CHAPTER 8

Conclusions and perspective

Contents

8.1 Major conclusions

Cyclospora cayetanensis was named by Ortega et al. in 1994 and has received further attention since the first outbreak of *Cyclospora*-associated diarrheal illness in the United States in 1990 (Huang et al., 1995; Ortega and Sanchez, 2010). Currently, a total of 22 *Cyclospora* species have been identified or described in vipers, moles, myriapodes, rodents, monkeys, and humans (Lainson, 2005; Li et al., 2015; McAllister et al., 2018). In addition, *Cyclospora*-like organisms have also been described in dogs, cattle, chickens, rats, house mice, birds, monkeys, shellfish, etc., and even in environmental samples (Sherchand and Cross, 2001; Chu et al., 2004; Li et al., 2007; Cordón et al., 2008; Aksoy et al., 2014; Helenbrook et al., 2015; Ghozzi et al., 2017). The presence of asexual and sexual stages in the same host suggests that the life cycle can be completed within one host (Ortega et al., 1997). Infection with *C. cayetanensis* is mainly transmitted through the ingestion of food contaminated with oocysts.

Small submit rRNA gene sequences show minimal genetic diversity among *C. cayetanensis* isolates from around the world (Sulaiman et al., 2014), and it is genetically related to members of the genus *Eimeria* (Relman et al., 1996). Phylogenetic analyses based on the mitochondrial and apicoplast genomes of *C. cayetanensis* have also confirmed the genetic similarities between *C. cayetanensis* and *Eimeria* spp. (Cinar et al., 2015; Ogedengbe et al., 2015; Tang et al., 2015; Liu et al., 2016). The whole genome of *C. cayetanensis* is estimated to have a total length of 44 Mbp, with 52% GC content and ~7500 gene (Liu et al., 2016). *C. cayetanensis* shares a coccidia-like metabolism and invasion components, but has unique surface antigens (Liu et al., 2016).

There are also some major differences in the amino acid metabolism and the posttranslational modification of proteins between *C. cayetanensis* and other apicomplexans (Liu et al., 2016).

At least 54 countries have documented *C. cayetanensis* infections (involving 13,845 cases) up to December 2018. Of these more than 13 have recorded cyclosporiasis outbreaks (including 6557 cases). The overall *C. cayetanensis* prevalence in humans worldwide is 3.55% (5478/154,410) (Li et al., 2020b). *C. cayetanensis* infections are commonly reported in developing countries with low-socioeconomic levels or disease-endemic areas, such as Madagascar, Nepal, Indonesia, Peru and Haiti, among others. However, large outbreaks have also been documented in developed countries in Europe and the Americas, and among travelers from these countries and those returning from tropical endemic areas (Li et al., 2020b). Among susceptible populations, the highest prevalence has been documented in immunocompetent individuals with diarrhea. The marked seasonality of *C. cayetanensis* infection, which occurs predominantly during the rainy season or summer, is well documented.

Detection methods based on oocyst morphology, staining, and molecular testing have been developed (Li et al., 2020a). Some new genotyping tools based on genomic data have been established (Barratt et al., 2019; Guo et al., 2019; Nascimento et al., 2019), which should be helpful in initial source-tracking studies and in distinguishing different case clusters, especially during cyclosporiasis outbreaks.

TMP-SMX has been proven effective treatment drug for human cyclosporiasis, and ciprofloxacin and nitazoxanide are the two alternative drugs (Li et al., 2020a). Magnesium oxide nanoparticles provide useful approach to prevent foodborne and waterborne contamination (Hussein et al., 2018). *Cyclospora* infections are frequently identified in travelers from areas of endemicity, thus these infections should therefore be considered in all travelers with diarrhea (Ortega and Sanchez, 2010). Adequate processing of water and foods and abstaining from consumption of raw produce when traveling to areas of endemicity will aid in reducing the risk of acquiring *Cyclospora* infection. Basic measures to prevent *Cyclospora* infection in humans include health education, correct personal hygiene, adequate hand washing, changes in eating habits, drinking boiled or bottled water and not eating raw produce, proper sanitary infrastructure, and the treatment of human sewage (Giangaspero and Gasser, 2019). In addition, good agricultural practices and use of filtered or otherwise decontaminated irrigation water should be implemented in countries where crops are grown for local consumption and exportation (Ortega and Sanchez, 2010). Moreover, food safety training worldwide is an absolutely necessity if progress is to be made in providing safe food and water to consumers internationally.

8.2 Perspective (future challenge)

There are many gaps in our knowledge of the epidemiology and other basic aspects of *C. cayetanensis* challenge our efforts to improve the knowledge of this protistan parasite and to prevent infections and disease. The widespread circulation of *C. cayetanensis* in humans, fresh produce, the environment, and in animals, means that there is a need for targeted action at different levels, in order to enable better understanding of this protozoan and to develop control strategies.

Routine tests for *C. cayetanensis* in clinical diagnostic laboratories are needed to further develop and optimize, because the accurate identification of the parasite species can facilitate rapid recovery. In addition, developing low cost, sensitive, and practical tests with broad applicability in developing countries is the future development direction, as well as developing "gold standard" molecular methods for rapid and reliable detection and diagnosis.

The number of genetic markers in current use is insufficient to reliably establish the extent of genetic diversity within and among *Cyclospora* populations from the same and distinct host animals. Therefore, there needs to be an increased focus on genomic studies of *Cyclospora* as a foundation for molecular, genetic, and epidemiological investigations, and the establishment of improved diagnostic and analytical tools using extensive panels of genetic markers. Moreover, genomic comparisons of different operational taxonomic units would lead to the identification of genes that are associated with their adaptation to different host species and enable the reliable differentiation of zoonotic from nonzoonotic taxa of *Cyclospora*. Such studies might also assist in identifying genes that are specific to zoonotic members of this genus and are essential for their survival, thus representing candidates for treatments, vaccines, or diagnostic targets. Progress in the genomics of *C. cayetanensis* has been slow, mainly because of the challenges in obtaining a sufficient amount of oocyst material, and the absence of in vitro cultivation and in vivo experimental infection systems. Therefore, several key areas relating biology could be focused on in the future, including developing in vitro and in vivo propagation systems, to study the pathogenesis at the cellular level, to ascertain the susceptibility of animals to *Cyclospora* and their roles as hosts or reservoirs of *C. cayetanensis*.

Surveillance is one of future collaborative researches needed on *Cyclospora*. Monitor treated irrigation and processed water, the efficiency of water treatment plants, and the correct use of manure as a fertilizer. Implement effective sanitary control of water used in agriculture, that is, irrigation of vegetables and fruits. Monitor wastewater treatment plant performance, use advanced inactivation technology in wastewater treatment plants. Develop new technologies for the removal or destruction of *Cyclospora* oocysts along the food chain, study the occurrence, distribution and fate of oocysts in the environment, estimate the level of disease risk, and evaluate the effectiveness of water treatment. Increase awareness of *Cyclospora* issues among food industry managers, key players in the food industry, food safety specialists, public health officials, and international food safety organizations.

References

Aksoy, U., Marangi, M., Papini, R., Ozkoc, S., Bayram Delibas, S., Giangaspero, A., 2014. Detection of *Toxoplasma gondii* and *Cyclospora cayetanensis* in *Mytilus galloprovincialis* from Izmir Province coast (Turkey) by real time PCR/high-resolution melting analysis (HRM). Food Microbiol. 44, 128–135.

Barratt, J.L.N., Park, S., Nascimento, F.S., Hofstetter, J., Plucinski, M., Casillas, S., Bradbury, R.S., Arrowood, M.J., Qvarnstrom, Y., Talundzic, E., 2019. Genotyping genetically heterogeneous *Cyclospora cayetanensis* infections to complement epidemiological case linkage. Parasitology 31, 1–33.

Chu, D.M., Sherchand, J.B., Cross, J.H., Orlandi, P.A., 2004. Detection of *Cyclospora cayetanensis* in animal fecal isolates from Nepal using an FTA filter-base polymerase chain reaction method. Am. J. Trop. Med. Hyg. 71, 373–379.

Cinar, H.N., Gopinath, G., Jarvis, K., Murphy, H.R., 2015. The complete mitochondrial genome of the foodborne parasitic pathogen *Cyclospora cayetanensis*. PLoS ONE 10, e0128645.

Cordón, G.P., Prados, A.H., Romero, D., Sánchez Moreno, M., Pontes, A., Osuna, A., Rosales, M.J., 2008. Intestinal parasitism in the animals of the zoological garden 'Peña Escrita' (Almuñecar, Spain). Vet. Parasitol. 156, 302–309.

Ghozzi, K., Marangi, M., Papini, R., Lahmar, I., Challouf, R., Houas, N., Ben Dhiab, R., Normanno, G., Babba, H., Giangaspero, A., 2017. First report of Tunisian coastal water contamination by protozoan parasites using mollusk bivalves as biological indicators. Mar. Pollut. Bull. 117, 197–202.

Giangaspero, A., Gasser, R.B., 2019. Human cyclosporiasis. Lancet Infect. Dis. 19, e226–e236.

Guo, Y., Wang, Y., Wang, X., Zhang, L., Ortega, Y., Feng, Y., 2019. Mitochondrial genome sequence variation as a useful marker for assessing genetic heterogeneity among *Cyclospora cayetanensis* isolates and source tracking. Parasit. Vectors 12, 47.

Helenbrook, W.D., Wade, S.E., Shields, W.M., Stehman, S.V., Whipps, C.M., 2015. Gastrointestinal parasites of Ecuadorian mantled howler monkeys (*Alouatta palliata aequatorialis*) based on fecal analysis. J. Parasitol. 101, 341–350.

Huang, P., Weber, J.T., Sosin, D.M., Griffin, P.M., Long, E.G., Murphy, J.J., Kocka, F., Peters, C., Kallick, C., 1995. The first reported outbreak of diarrheal illness associated with *Cyclospora* in the United States. Ann. Intern. Med. 123, 409–414.

Hussein, E.M., Ahmed, S.A., Mokhtar, A.B., Elzagawy, S.M., Yahi, S.H., Hussein, A.M., El-Tantawey, F., 2018. Antiprotozoal activity of magnesium oxide (MgO) nanoparticles against *Cyclospora cayetanensis* oocysts. Parasitol. Int. 67, 666–674.

Lainson, R., 2005. The genus *Cyclospora* (apicomplexa: Eimeriidae), with a description of *Cyclospora schneideri* n. sp. in the snake Anilius scytale scytale (Aniliidae) from Amazonian Brazil—a review. Mem. Inst. Oswaldo Cruz 100, 103–110.

Li, G., Xiao, S., Zhou, R., Li, W., Wadeh, H., 2007. Molecular characterization of *Cyclospora*-like organism from dairy cattle. Parasitol. Res. 100, 955–961.

Li, N., Ye, J., Arrowood, M.J., Ma, J., Wang, L., Xu, H., Feng, Y., Xiao, L., 2015. Identification and morphologic and molecular characterization of *Cyclospora macacae* n. sp. from rhesus monkeys in China. Parasitol. Res. 114, 1811–1816.

Li, J., Cui, Z., Qi, M., Zhang, L., 2020a. Advances in *Cyclosporiasis* diagnosis and therapeutic intervention. Front. Cell. Infect. Microbiol. 10, 43.

Li, J., Wang, R., Chen, Y., Xiao, L., Zhang, L., 2020b. *Cyclospora cayetanensis* infection in humans: biological characteristics, clinical features, epidemiology, detection method and treatment. Parasitology 147, 160–170.

Liu, S., Wang, L., Zheng, H., Xu, Z., Roellig, D.M., Li, N., Frace, M.A., Tang, K., Arrowood, M.J., Moss, D.M., Zhang, L., Feng, Y., Xiao, L., 2016. Comparative genomics reveals *Cyclospora cayetanensis* possesses coccidialike metabolism and invasion components but unique surface antigens. BMC Genomics 17, 316.

McAllister, C.T., Motriuk-Smith, D., Kerr, C.M., 2018. Three new coccidians (*Cyclospora*, *Eimeria*) from eastern moles, *Scalopus aquaticus* (Linnaeus) (Mammalia: Soricomorpha: Talpidae) from Arkansas, USA. Syst. Parasitol. 95, 271–279.

Nascimento, F.S., Barta, J.R., Whale, J., Hofstetter, J.N., Casillas, S., Barratt, J., Talundzic, E., Arrowood, M.J., Qvarnstrom, Y., 2019. Mitochondrial junction region as genotyping marker for *Cyclospora cayetanensis*. Emerg. Infect. Dis. 25, 1314–1319.

Ogedengbe, M.E., Qvarnstrom, Y., da Silva, A.J., Arrowood, M.J., Barta, J.R., 2015. A linear mitochondrial genome of *Cyclospora cayetanensis* (Eimeriidae, Eucoccidiorida, Coccidiasina, Apicomplexa) suggests the ancestral start position within mitochondrial genomes of *Eimeriid coccidia*. Int. J. Parasitol. 45, 361–365.

Ortega, Y.R., Sanchez, R., 2010. Update on *Cyclospora cayetanensis*, a foodborne and waterborne parasite. Clin. Microbiol. Rev. 23, 218–234.

Ortega, Y.R., Nagle, R., Gilman, R.H., Watanabe, J., Miyagui, J., Quispe, H., Kanagusuku, P., Roxas, C., Sterling, C.R., 1997. Pathologic and clinical findings in patients with cyclosporiasis and a description of intracellular parasite life-cycle stages. J Infect Dis 176, 1584–1589.

Relman, D.A., Schmidt, T.M., Gajadhar, A., Sogin, M., Cross, J., Yoder, K., Sethabutr, O., Echeverria, P., 1996. Molecular phylogenetic analysis of *Cyclospora*, the human intestinal pathogen, suggests that it is closely related to *Eimeria* species. J. Infect. Dis. 173, 440–445.

Sherchand, J.B., Cross, J.H., 2001. Emerging pathogen *Cyclospora cayetanensis* infection in Nepal. Southeast Asian J. Trop. Med. Public Health 32, 143–150.

Sulaiman, I.M., Ortega, Y., Simpson, S., Kerdahi, K., 2014. Genetic characterization of human-pathogenic *Cyclospora cayetanensis* parasites from three endemic regions at the 18S ribosomal RNA locus. Infect. Genet. Evol. 22, 229–234.

Tang, K., Guo, Y., Zhang, L., Rowe, L.A., Roellig, D.M., Frace, M.A., Li, N., Liu, S., Feng, Y., Xiao, L., 2015. Genetic similarities between *Cyclospora cayetanensis* and cecum-infecting avian *Eimeria* spp. in apicoplast and mitochondrial genomes. Parasit. Vectors 8, 358.

Index

Note: Page numbers followed by *f* indicate figures and *t* indicate tables.

Enzyme-linked immunosorbent assay-based
OLA, 141
Enzyme-linked immunosorbent assay
(ELISA) method, 142–143
Extraintestinal infection, 49–51

F

Faculty of Tropical Medicine, 48–49
Fecal-oral transmission cycle, 150
Flow cytometry, 137–138
Food sample contamination, 125–129,
126–128*t*
Fresh unfixed oocysts, 136

G

Gastrointestinal disease, 57. *See also* Biliary
disease
Gastrointestinal symptoms, 136
GBS. *See* Guillain-Barre syndrome (GBS)
Genome characteristics
apicoplast genome, 38–39
chromosome genome, 39–40
mitochondrial genome, 36–38
Ghost oocysts, 138–139
Glomeris (Diplopoda), 2
"Gold standard" molecular methods,
157
Good agricultural practices, 156–157
Guillain-Barre syndrome (GBS), 50

H

HAART, 148–150
Histopathological findings, 51
Host, 2–3, 4–6*t*, 21–22, 26–28
Human cyclosporiasis, 28, 104–105, 121,
135. *See also* Cyclosporiasis
epidemiological determinants and risk
factors for, 129*t*
outbreaks of, 58, 63–65*t*
pathogenic organism, 2
Human immune state, 98
Humans, 148, 151
Cyclospora cayetanensis in, 34–35, 58–98,
59*f*, 60–62*t*
Cyclospora detected in, 7–8
cyclosporiasis case reports in, 87–97*t*
Hygiene and sanitary condition, *Cyclospora
cayetanensis* infection, 100

I

Immunofluorescent-antibody (IFA)
microscopy, 142–143
Internal transcribed spacer (ITS)
sequences, 34
Intestinal infection, 46–49
Intracytoplasmic development, 3
Intranuclear coccidiosis, 49
In vitro infectivity models, 150–151
In vitro methods, 151
In vivo methods, 151
ITS sequences. *See* Internal transcribed
spacer (ITS) sequences

J

Jejunal biopsies, 52

K

Kimura 2-parameter model, 37*f*

L

Lamina propria, in duodenum, 51–52
Life cycle, 2–3, 10
of *Cyclospora*, 26–28
Light microscopy, 8–9

M

Magnesium oxide (MgO) nanoparticles,
152, 156–157
Marked seasonality transmissions, 122
Metadata analysis, 47–48
Microscopic detection, of oocysts, 136
Microscopy, 136–137
Mitochondrial genome, 36–38
Mixed inflammatory cell infiltration, 52
MLM. *See* Myelin-like material (MLM)
MLST tool. *See* Multilocus sequence typing
(MLST) tool
Modified safranin technique, 139
Mogera wogura coreana, 2–3
Molecular-based detection methods,
34–35
Molecular characteristics, 33
case-linking and tracking, 41
genome characteristics, 36–40
of main loci, 34–36
Molecular diagnostic method, 34–35
Molecular genotyping, 41

Printed in the United States
by Baker & Taylor Publisher Services